Alycia Oppenheim has a bachelor's degree from the University of South Florida and a master's degree in Shakespeare Studies from the Shakespeare Institute in England. Passionate about social change, Alycia strives to make a difference in the world. While not working at her full-time job, Alycia is an adjunct professor of English Composition.

Dr. Phyllis Oppenheim holds a doctorate in health sciences from Nova Southeastern and a master's degree in health services administration. Because of Alycia's struggle with eating disorders, her doctorate focus was eating disorders in general and, specifically, both the early warning signs of an eating disorder and spreading awareness of them.

To say that I dedicate this book to everyone I have met along my journey seems ridiculous, as there are many whose paths I crossed during this journey that had no influence on my struggles or, unintentionally, hurt me. However, there are many who have helped shape the person I have become, and it is to them I dedicate this book.

Without my "Frew" (Renfrew) girls, I would have been lost in a period of time when the darkness seemed to be overwhelming. Throughout the years, you girls have given me the type of love and understanding that others are incapable of giving. We have shared meals, tears, stories, laughter, and overwhelming vulnerability. It was with each of you that I was able to show the true me, even at my darkest times, and I know that I have a friend in each of you. I cherish and love you all, and I dedicate this book to you.

No battle can be fought without its army, and my family has been the greatest army anyone could have. At times it has been difficult, and I know it has not been easy. However, they have continued to stand by my side and fight through all of the demons, not just ED. My family has shown me what it means to love unconditionally and with unwavering devotion. It is to them I dedicate this book.

ED does not make it easy to date. ED does not make it easy for me to be loved, or at least I do not think so. But, for five years, one person overlooked my shadow and stuck through it all with me. This person—who stood on the battlefield, on the front lines and through tears and fights, through cuts and all the other battle wounds—still found ways to love me. This person shared my meal plans, went to groups, spent nights in hospitals and days in treatment centers. He saw me at my lowest and still held me on the highest of pedestals. This person showed me what it felt like to be loved as a person, not as a sick girl, and he will always hold a special place in my heart. It is to him that I dedicate this book.

To my "Frew" girls, my family, and to the man from my past, thank you. Thank you for drying my tears. Thank you for never giving up on me. Thank you for being in groups, for listening to my therapists when I don't or didn't. Thank you for helping me believe in me, instead of letting me believe in ED.

-Alycia Oppenheim

Alycia and Phyllis Oppenheim

ED: MY SHADOW, NOT MY FRIEND

AUSTIN MACAULEY PUBLISHERS™

LONDON · CAMBRIDGE · NEW YORK · SHARJAH

Ordering Information:
Quantity sales: special discounts are available on quantity purchases by corporations, associations, and others. For details, contact the publisher at the address below.

Publisher's Cataloguing-in-Publication data
Oppenheim, Alycia and Oppenheim, Phyllis
ED: My Shadow, Not My Friend

ISBN 9781645363934 (Paperback)
ISBN 9781645363927 (Hardback)
ISBN 9781645363958 (ePub e-book)

Library of Congress Control Number: 2020900795

www.austinmacauley.com/us

First Published (2020)
Austin Macauley Publishers LLC
40 Wall Street, 28th Flo
New York, NY 10005
USA

mail-usa@austinmacauley.com
+1 (646) 5125767

Author's Note

I have tried to recreate events, locales and conversations from my memories of them. In order to maintain their anonymity in some instances, I have changed the names of individuals and places; I may have changed some identifying characteristics and details such as physical properties, occupations and places of residence. Austin Macaulay Publishers will not be liable for any and all claims or causes of action, known or unknown, arising out of the contents of this book.

To those who told me I couldn't succeed, I thrived.

To Lachi, for giving me strength and to Zeidi (grandfather) for giving me wisdom, without both of you, I would not have been able to fight my shadow.

To Greg, Dad and Mom, thanks for never giving up.

A Mother's Acknowledgments

There are many people who have been a part of or a party to our family's journey with Aly's eating disorder. Some of these individuals were a positive part of our journey while others, were negative. However, it is said that there is a positive in every negative (or, a silver lining in every cloud). I believe that to be true.

For that reason, I would like to acknowledge the psychologists, school administrators, principals, and teachers who failed so miserably with Aly. Whether by not identifying her issues early enough to help her avoid this journey or by failing to help us understand what was happening, or by telling her that she could not accomplish her dreams, these individuals failed. However, many of their failures might have been the impetus for our move to Florida; a move that, I believe, helped Aly to ultimately become the incredible woman that she is today.

On the other side, I want to acknowledge my father who passed away before seeing Aly mature and accomplish so much and his life companion who has also passed away. Having these two people in our lives during many parts of this journey provided incredible support and strength. We miss both of them every day but know that they are always watching over us.

I also want to acknowledge Jeff, my amazing husband and Aly's father and Greg, my incredible son and Aly's brother. The journey has been difficult on all of us but throughout, they have provided strength and, at times, laughter in the face of so much pain. Together, we have gotten past so much and seen the shadow of Aly's ED dissipate. Thank you so much.

Table of Contents

I lay on the floor, feeling the bathroom tile under my back
as the cold rushes through me,
The taste of vomit still in my mouth.
I don't know how I got back here.

I don't know how I'm back at the point with the grasp so
tight around me.
Everything feels so numb and yet I can feel sharp feelings
of pain
Tremble through me like small earthquakes beneath my
skin.

It feels like I'm remembering another person when I think
of days filled with smiles, laughter, and love.
Am I the same girl who fled the grasp of her captor just to
be back once again?

Nothing makes sense anymore and as I lay here staring up
at the starless ceiling, I wonder if anything ever will again.

Introduction

It all began with no warning. Like the start of the world, one day there was nothing and then slowly things began appearing. One day I just remember thinking of imperfections. There was a line here or a piece of fat there and then it was all of me; all of me was imperfect and all of me needed to change. I would look around at the other girls around me and think of whether they would wake up in the morning and look at themselves to pick out their imperfections. Probably not. I thought I was different. I thought I was strange. I didn't fit in. As time went on, I remember the voice joining the equation.

The next addition to the creation of my world was the sound of this little voice in my head telling me everything was going to be okay and that it had all of the answers. That voice was my friend. That voice was what kept me going when I felt alone in the realization that I was different from everyone else around me. I didn't need to be like everyone else as long as I had that voice telling me everything was going to be okay. The voice would tell me of my imperfections but would tell me of ways to cure the imperfections. Then came the next steps. Next was restriction. Restriction was the piece of the puzzle that started to make the picture. I started to see what I could be or what the voice wanted me to see. After restriction came the purging and then the laxatives until the whole world was created. My ED world was created, and I lived in that world. I thought I thrived in that world. I thought I needed that world. I lived in that world for years until that world created a new world. That world created a world of doctors, pain, medicine, bed rest, sadness, and confusion. My ED world became confusing and damaged. It was nothing like what I thought it would be and that picture that began forming when I was young was a mirage. It was a lie that ED made up to keep me trapped. This is the story of the creation of my ED world.

I've been living with my eating disorder for over 18 years. I don't have memories of life before ED's voice became a part of my day-to-day life. I didn't know what it was at first. The voice started off quiet, like a wind brushing by my ear and then became louder than my own voice. As my body changed when I was younger, so did how I viewed myself. I wanted to look like the other girls in my class. Even at a young age I would compare myself to the other people around me and wonder why I wasn't like them. I was sad and lonely the majority of the time.

At 29, there are times that I feel sad that I still feel like I did at 10. Every day brings a different trial, a different thought; a different comparison. Some days are easier than others. I can get through all my meals with very few negative thoughts. Other days it is hard getting out of bed and even harder to convince myself that it is a good idea to put food in my system.

Having my ED in my head makes my thoughts unclear and causes me to jump to conclusions. Sometimes, I'll think of eating a meal and my ED will go from "you shouldn't eat that" to "if you eat that then you'll gain weight and if you gain weight then no one will love you and if no one will love you then you'll die alone and then no one will miss you when you go." All of this comes out of eating a piece of fruit or some nuts. When I look in the mirror, it is like looking in a circus mirror. People tell me I look "healthy" and that I am beautiful, but I don't see that. I see disgust and fatness and sadness. Sometimes, I stand in front of the mirror and I just look at myself and try and pick out things that I could learn to like. It doesn't work once I get past my eyes. I hate what I see in the mirror and with those negative thoughts, the idea intrudes that there is an easy way to get rid of all that I hate, and I begin purging or restricting. Logically, I know that neither of those options are good ways to lose weight and that by eating healthy and exercising I could get to a HEALTHY weight instead of a sick weight. However, my mind doesn't think like that and each day I still struggle. It is in these times when my logical mind is supposed to help me, when my logical mind should make sense.

Life has never been easy when it comes to my eating disorder and, unfortunately, the warning signs at a young age were ignored because eating disorders weren't spoken about back then. My elementary school teacher informed my parents that they didn't see me eat; that I was skipping meals. My parent's response was that I just wasn't hungry, and our lives went on as they had before they were told. I would skip certain meals and they would continue to have their heads in the sand. I don't blame my parents for ED coming into my life. I don't think that there was anything they could have done then except maybe share more body-positive thoughts. ED found its way into my mind and has lived there most of my life and the only thing to blame is the eating disorder itself; to blame this mental disease that has burrowed its way into my life, into my very being.

Throughout the years, I've spent in and out of treatment, I have learned a lot of coping mechanisms, words of advice, etc. Unfortunately, it is easy to listen to someone tell you what to do and even harder to implement those coping mechanisms into your own life. It is sometimes easy to listen to someone tell you the best way to do something, even the best way to recover, but they don't live in your shoes and they don't know what brought you to where your path has taken you; they can't tell you what works best for you. Sometimes, it takes a long time to figure out the best way to do something for you and not for other people.

It's taken me a long time to figure out what works for me and what doesn't. Some days, some things work and the next day that same thing may not. I spent almost two years in recovery, thanks to someone that I loved very much, using him as my own personal coping mechanism. However, when he left, I was left alone to figure out what things worked for me all over again and there were many days that I felt that I was not strong enough or that I didn't want to fight anymore. I used that person as a coping mechanism because it worked for me most of the time; it was the one thing that kept pushing me forward to do better or to be better. That was something that I knew I could count on when I was at my lowest. But then, when I got to my lowest and he wasn't there, I was left with nothing. Trauma has a tendency to push me more towards ED rather than trying to fight in honor of someone else that I've lost or has left me.

The purpose of this book is not just to talk about eating disorders, but to also talk about what life is like from two different perspectives; one, from me who lives with the eating disorder on a daily basis, and one, from my mom and other family members that have chosen to support me throughout my fight. My brother once told me that he would be willing to fight by my side and go through hell beside me, but that he couldn't fight this fight without me; that this is my battle and he is just my lieutenant.

My hope for this book is to not only show what it is like to live with the eating disorder as well as life with a loved one with an eating disorder, but also to help families get on the front lines and fight beside their daughters and sons. No matter how strong we may look on the outside, this disease isolates us from those we love. The best way to strike a blow against ED is to bring people in and let them help. Sometimes it gets difficult and sometimes, your loved one just wants to scream and tell someone struggling to just stop and eat, but it is so much more than that. Those struggling need patience and love. They need as much understanding as you can give having not lived with this disease yourself. This is a deadly disease. It kills more people every year than any other mental illness and it has become a pandemic that insurance companies and the government want to ignore. It is up to us to fight and the best way to start is to understand the monster that we are dealing with and how it affects the people that surround us. Throughout this book I will refer to my demon, my eating disorder as ED. At times, ED may also be referred to as him, he, his, or it. You may have a different name for your eating disorder, but mine has always had the voice of a male and I have named him ED. So, here is my journey and the journey of my family. I hope this helps and makes a difference on your front line and anyone you share this with.

October 2018

A Mother's Introduction

Even before our children are born, our prayers and dreams are for them to grow up healthy and strong; to be able to provide for them in every way possible; to help them mature so that they can one day fly away. From the moment that they enter the world, we instinctively want to protect them; to hold them close and shield them from harm or pain. Unfortunately, no matter how fervently we pray, no matter how hard we try, there are some demons that infiltrate their lives and the world changes.

This is what happened to our family. It did not happen overnight and once it begins, there is no real end. We pray that our precious daughter will find herself permanently in recovery but know that, unlike strep throat or pneumonia or a thousand other diseases, for many, life becomes a vicious cycle of recovery and relapse. Similar to alcoholism and drug abuse, those afflicted live their lives at risk for relapsing and their families and friends must always be vigilant and strong with their support and love.

Our nightmare began years before we recognized the demon for what it is. Eating disorders, which we shall refer to by the name "ED" throughout, have a way of creeping into your life. We did not know the warning signs; did not know the red flags. Even when one of her teachers reached out to express concern that our daughter was not eating, we were in total denial. We were sure that it was just part of adolescence and nothing to be concerned with. God, I wish I knew then what I know now. And, that is why I am writing this for our daughter's book. Parents must learn the warning signs, must know the red flags. Parents must also not be ashamed of the possibility that their sons or daughters have an eating disorder. It is nothing to be ashamed of; the shame is in doing nothing about it.

It took years for us to face her reality, to recognize that Aly had an eating disorder. Years that could have been avoided had we known back then what we know now. Years of suffering that she might not have had to face. But 18 years ago, even 15 years ago, pediatricians were not suggesting the possibility of an eating disorder. Early puberty was not considered a predictor or possible warning sign of what the future might hold. Unfortunately, this is true even today. Most health care professionals receive little if any education on eating disorders. What training they might get is woefully limited. Between the lack of awareness, the lack of insurance coverage, the lack of legislation to help these boys and girls, men and women, millions suffer every day, many do not receive treatment, and many die.

We are sharing our ED journey to help other families recognize the early warning signs of eating disorders. We are sharing our ED journey in hopes that telling our story will prevent other young women and men from having to travel down this terrible road. And, we are sharing our ED journey in hopes of removing the stigma that surrounds eating disorders. Anorexia, bulimia, binge eating disorder are illnesses; illnesses for which there are no cures, no vaccines. These illnesses are killers of dreams, of hopes, and lives.

October 2018

Chapter 1

Over 30 million men and women in the
United States struggle with eating disorders.[1]

Memories of a Mother

One of the happiest days of our lives was learning that I was pregnant with our second child. The pregnancy was great but lasted almost three weeks longer than anticipated. Even then, Aly was demonstrating her stubbornness and head-strong need to do things when she was ready and not a moment sooner. Unfortunately, her arrival was terrifying, to say the least.

We arrived at the hospital after laboring at home most of the day. Thankfully, I was fully dilated on arrival and Aly was in a hurry to make her entrance. Less than 30 minutes after arriving at the hospital, Aly made her entrance. Not like most babies, crying and pink. Her umbilical cord was wrapped around her neck several times and she was cyanotic and not breathing. Those first few moments waiting to hear her cry, were the worst moments of our lives. Thank God for the nurses and doctors who rushed to her aid, resuscitated her, and assured us that she would be okay.

Perhaps, her first day of life was her first day of her eating disorder. We will never know, but over the years I have thought about it. The day after she was born (the remainder of that first day she spent in the NICU being monitored to be sure she continued breathing), the nurse brought her to me to nurse. No luck. My precious, beautiful daughter was obviously hungry but would not nurse. She would also not take a bottle.

The second day, we tried again. This time, a wonderful nurse sat with me and explained that Aly's throat was scratched during the resuscitation efforts, so it was hard for her to swallow. She showed me how to hold her so that she could take the formula from a bottle with a neonatal nipple. We had to hold her in such a way that she was almost sitting straight but, in doing so, at least she could and would eat.

We brought her home after three nights in the hospital. On day 4, we learned what projectile vomiting was. It seemed that she was throwing up as much as she was taking in. The pediatrician assured us that was not the case and, he must have been right. At two weeks, we took her to the pediatrician, and she had gained a little weight, despite not eating well the first few days and despite her vomiting several times a day.

Life with Aly settled down a bit after that. She was a great sleeper and slept through the night at six weeks. Her smile lit up her whole face and no one who saw that smile could resist smiling with her. Aly's big blue eyes and amazing smile brought joy to so many. She also melted hearts so much that, at about three months, my father was watching me play with Aly. It was that day that he said to me: "She is manipulating you already, Phyllis. Watch that little one. She already has you and Jeff wrapped around her little finger." You know, he was absolutely right.

Did those early days of her life set the stage for what was to come? In my saner moments I don't think so, but in those dark nights when sleep eludes me, the mind starts to question everything. When did ED intrude in our lives? Was ED always lurking behind the scenes? Did her early days of not eating and purging somehow affect her as she reached adolescence? There are no answers to these questions, but we would, eventually, learn answers to other questions.

***I thought of all of my flaws when I looked in the mirror
and with those thoughts, I hated what I saw.***

– Alycia Oppenheim

Dear Diary,

I wish I lived in the movies. Then I would be beautiful. Sometimes, I like to pretend that I am in the movies so that just for a second, I can make myself believe that I don't look the way that I do. I can bat my eyes and smile and pretend that I am the leading lady and that boys will look at me. Then I come back and remember that I am not the leading lady. I am fat. I hate my body. I don't look like the other girls in my class. They are so much prettier than me and everyone knows it. I don't know what to do with myself. I skip breakfast sometimes and I think that makes me feel better. I don't know why that makes me feel better, but it does.

I don't tell anyone anything, but maybe, if I tell one of my best friends, they could help. I'd probably sound crazy telling them I have a voice in my head. They wouldn't understand. It isn't a crazy voice in my head. I'm not insane. I just know somehow that not eating breakfast is the right thing to do because maybe it will help me lose weight and then I will be beautiful. There is this soft whisper that tells me this is the right thing; like a conscience leading me down the right path telling me that if I don't eat, I will be happy.

I feel sad a lot of the time. No one notices. No one cares. I wish people cared. Don't I? I think I want people to care about me, but I also want people to leave me alone. No one knows what it is like to be like me. No one knows what it is like to live in my body and to think the way that I do. I hate myself. I wish I looked like the other girls. I wish I was looked at the way that they are looked at and I wasn't so weird.

Sincerely,
Sad, little Care Bear.
(circa 2000)

I spent my childhood comparing myself to everyone around me. Why wasn't I as thin as the other girls? Why did they get more attention than me? Why was my body changing and their bodies were staying the same? I wanted so badly to fit in or at least feel like I fit in. Even before I can remember comparing myself to the girls around me, I still wasn't happy with my body.

When I was little, I used to cut the hair off of my Barbies and make them look ugly so that I didn't feel inferior to them. It sounds sick and sad, but even at that young of an age, there was something about me that I hated; that wasn't good enough. As my body began changing and I started becoming a "woman," I tried doing what women do in the movies and use it to get attention. I would bat my eyelashes and throw my head back when I laughed. I figured that maybe I'd fit in if the boys liked me, but the problem was that the more attention that I got, the less the other girls liked me. I was pushed further out of the circle than I was before.

I spent a lot of time during my youth just trying to feel like I fit in and belonged somewhere. Even at a young age, I felt that something was missing. As I have gotten older, I have found ways to deal with that missing part of me, but when I was little and feeling left out I spent my time trying to change my body, while simultaneously, putting scars all over my skin.

Self-harming began to be a part of my day-to-day life. It was a way for me to control the only thing I had control over: pain. I didn't realize that I was already gaining some control by not eating. ED hadn't made himself fully known at that point. It took many years for me to realize what the sound in the back of my head was; to acknowledge that there was a separate part of me. There was an evil part that was trying to kill me; a shadow that was following me and taunting me. I didn't realize until I was much older that I was letting that side of me control every move I was making.

ED has always had a way of controlling me even before I realized what it was. I spent most of my life believing that I was in control. I believed that it was my choices that were brought about by what others did to me. I spent a lot of time blaming others for my hurting myself. The sad part is that I used those people, even my family, to convince myself that it was okay to hurt myself. I feel like when I was younger, I wanted to hurt those around me because I was so angry and hurt. I felt ignored and lonely all the time. I felt alone and ignored even when I was at the table having dinner with my family. There were so many thoughts screaming inside my head that I couldn't turn off or tell anyone. I lived in a haze all around me that I felt no one could possibly understand. It wasn't until I was older that I learned that the haze was caused by being bipolar and by depression.

There is a saying that I was told in treatment that "you are only as sick as your secrets" and it couldn't have been truer. I kept everything to myself. All my fears and insecurities, I let live inside my head or in the cuts and scars on my arms and legs. I let my insecurities lead what I did. I did stupid things all the time to get attention; to make myself believe that people cared about me. Looking at it now, it was all superficial. I would make guys do things; manipulate them in order to make myself feel special. When I think about it now, I wasn't a very nice person and that is one of my only regrets in my 28 years of life. To be honest, I do not know what came first, my insecurities or my ED. Now I know that doesn't make sense. The logical response is that I was insecure and that led the way for ED. I remember missing meals before I remember being insecure and having low self-esteem. My eating disorder was more than just a disease. From a young age, it became my way of life; it was how I survived. To be completely honest, I remember the pain. The pain is what came before everything and that is what I think led to ED and the insecurities.

When I was younger, it felt like my body would shut down sometimes. I felt like the closer I got to a three-digit weight, the worse I would get. I would stop eating and cry and stop getting hungry; sometimes I would purge. I felt like getting to three digits meant that everything in my world would end; it was life altering the closer that I would get. I can honestly say that growing up after ED entered my life, my greatest fear was gaining weight. I couldn't give in to the weight and the food even if it took my life. Being small and skinny and, what I thought was pretty, was worth more than anything else; anyone else.

Something that also impacted how I saw the world and myself was the first time I had a glimpse of what ED could do if you upset him. When I was younger, I had a best friend. She was the world to me. She meant more to me than best friends should as my world revolved around her. My friend had an awful childhood and used ED and self-harming as a way to cope with the tragedies of her life. I would sit in the attic bedroom with her and hold the towel on her arm when she would bleed. I sat in the room and watched television or read when she spent time in the bathroom. We spent our time talking about all these things that hurt her.

One day, I found out that she wasn't at home anymore. They took her to the hospital in order to help her with her eating disorder. ED had won the battle. My best friend was in the hospital because she couldn't survive life without the help of the doctors anymore. My mom took me to visit her in the hospital one time. We had made a deal that if I started eating, she would take me to see my friend in the hospital. This is when I started purging. It was like I was seeing someone that I didn't know. She didn't look like my best friend anymore. I looked into her eyes and they were dark brown pits with no light in them. I didn't know what to do, but it scared me. It didn't scare me out of ED, but it scared me out of that hospital. I promised myself that I would have more control and that I wouldn't let the disorder consume me like it did her. I didn't understand what happens when you let ED control your life. Even seeing her in the hospital like that didn't stop me. All it did was teach me that ED is who you listen to. She must have done something to upset it and that is why she was there. Even today more than a decade later, I can still see the hospital visiting area, my friend and those empty brown eyes. Even today they still scare me, but ED still scares me more.

Memories of a Mother

Despite our terrifying first moments and early months worrying about Aly, life moved on and she thrived. Adored by her big brother, father, grandfather, and great grandfather, Aly had a wonderful childhood. She was a happy, precocious child; inquisitive and incredibly articulate. Once Aly started talking, there was no stopping her. With her expanding vocabulary and apparent love of being in the center of it all, Aly demonstrated her fearlessness, lack of shyness, and desire to teach, even at a very young age.

In 1994, my father took all of us to Israel. Aly was not yet four years old. The second day of our trip was Friday and Aly and her older brother, Greg, met their first cousins for the first time. Many three-year-old children would be shy and stay close to their parents. Not our Aly. That Friday evening was the second time that Aly scared us beyond belief. I had thought that her birth was the most frightening time of my life. That was until my little girl disappeared from the hotel in Jerusalem and no one knew where she was. Thankfully, she had gone with her first cousins (who she had just met and who did not speak a word of English) to the synagogue. Terrifying moments that, thankfully, like those minutes in the birthing room not even four years earlier, ended quickly and she was safe and fine.

On the return flight, Aly disappeared on the plane. Hard to imagine, how you can lose your child on a trans-Atlantic flight but, trust me, it is possible. She had been playing on the floor in the bulkhead, Jeff was watching a movie, Greg was playing his Game Boy, and I was reading. Suddenly, no Aly. We found her rather quickly (she couldn't go too far on an airplane). She was in the galley, teaching the flight attendants how to tie their shoes. She spent almost the entire 12 hours of the flight in the galley with the flight attendants and crew. They loved our blonde hair, blue-eyed, articulate, and precocious angel and, of course, so did we.

Less than a year after the shoe-tying class given on El Al, Aly decided that she wanted to look like me, that she did not like the way she looked. So, Aly being Aly, she took matters into her own hands and proceeded to cut off her ponytail. The beautiful blonde curls were gone, left in a pile on the floor of her room. (I still have those blonde locks in a freezer bag in my file cabinet.) Thankfully, she did not do a bad job and our beautician friend was able to even out her hair and style it. This incident was a red flag, a red flag that we did not recognize then and did not recognize as a concern until many years later. Children should not hate the way they look at that age. Little children should not think of themselves as fat or ugly. Four-year old children should not be trying to change their appearance. I don't know why she felt that way then and I have never understood this. Aly was a child that was constantly being told how pretty she was, how beautiful her eyes were, how pretty her smile. Why then did she not see that? Had I been able to ask that question then and get answers, maybe her future would have been different. But I didn't ask the questions then and, by the time I knew enough to question this behavior, it was too late. ED had taken control like a parasitic leach that controlled her thoughts.

In kindergarten, Aly again demonstrated her stubbornness and determination. I spent many nights helping my children with homework, drilling them on consonants or vowel signs. I knew that Aly knew everything that she was being taught in school. That is why we were shocked when we received a phone call from her kindergarten teachers. They were concerned that she was not learning, was not participating, and surprised that she could not tie her own shoes. We were astounded by both pronouncements since we knew she knew her consonants and vowels and everyone on El Al knew two years earlier that she could tie her shoes. So, what was going on?

After meeting with her teachers, Jeff and I sat down with our daughter and told her what the teachers said. We asked her what was going on. Why was she not raising her hand or answering questions and why did she tell them that she could not tie her shoes? With incredible clarity and her blue eyes opened wide, with her hands on her hips she told us why. She said, "Mom, it's their fault. I raised my hand. A lot of times to answer questions. They never called on me, so I stopped raising my hand."

And why, Aly, did you tell them you could not tie your shoes?

"Oh, mommy, that's simple. I wanted to tie the boys' shoes and they wouldn't let me. So, I thought that they didn't

want to know that I knew how." Very simple. Very matter-of-fact.

At the risk of our daughter failing kindergarten, we came up with a plan that, thankfully, her teachers went along with. We suggested that they let Aly "teach" the class. That would demonstrate to them that Aly knew the material. It would also help Aly feel good about herself. The plan worked, and Aly demonstrated that, in fact, she knew all of the material. She was promoted to 1st grade.

From first through fourth grade, life settled down. There were hiccups and struggles but, for the most part, life moved on and both Aly and her brother continued to grow up and mature. Those years flew by and Aly was suddenly heading to middle school (grade 5 in the school she attended) and, shockingly, Aly also became a woman. Puberty came when she just turned 10, several years before most of her friends. Looking back, this was when ED began to exert control over Aly. This was when, in my opinion, Aly's dislike of her appearance began in earnest and early puberty helped to propel her down a spiraling path to self-hate, lack of self-esteem, and destructive behaviors.

Chapter 2

Every 62 minutes, at least one person dies as the direct result of an eating disorder.[2]

Fear the Hand That Hurts You.
– Alycia Oppenheim

Puberty is never easy for anyone. Your body is changing, and you are going through feelings that you think that no one can understand, except for you. I started puberty when I was 10, so I was right when I felt that no one around me could relate to what I was experiencing. Once again, I was different. That ED voice kept telling me that because my body was changing, I had to do more things to make it so I looked like the other girls.

When I got to middle school, everything was different. I had my ED and I was self-harming. People would see the cuts on my arms or my legs and stare at me. No one knew, how to handle what I was. I was "a cutter" or I was crazy, and I needed more help than they were willing or able to offer. The therapists at the school would even look at me strangely when I would try and talk to them about the pain I was feeling. I was always visiting their office or missing class to go to the nurse's office. Something always hurt; I was always in pain. The pain was something that was hidden deep inside of me. It stalked around the halls in my shadow. People could see it if they looked hard enough, but it was as if it was a glimpse of something that wasn't worth focusing on.

I was one of the poster children for my school. You would see my picture in their newsletter and when you walked in the door. My face would be right there with my bright blue/grey eyes and blonde hair. I always had a big smile on my face to make it look like my school was the happiest place to be. No one saw the troubled girl behind those smiles.

I spent a lot of time in school being called derogatory names. I don't know if anyone in my class knew what they meant, but the most common one was "slut" or a "ho." I used this as ammunition to hurt myself. I would write "ho" into my leg and cry as I would remember that the people I called friends were the ones saying this stuff behind my back. The worst part was that a part of me felt that I deserved it. I've spent so much of my life believing I deserve all of the bad things that happen to me and yet I never know why that is. I've even said the words over the years "I deserved what happened to me," but I never have a reason when someone asks me why. I know that when I was younger, I would do things with boys to get attention. I wanted so badly to be liked; for people to want to be around me, but I didn't know how to accomplish that. I made mistakes, but did that mean I deserved the vicious and hurtful names they called me or the way I was treated?

Before the end of the first half of 7th grade, some horrible events occurred that changed who I was. I was suspended from school and ultimately expelled from that "happy place." I was suspended for supposedly bringing a knife to school. They never found the knife (because there was no knife), but because of the cuts on my arms and several students said they saw a knife, I was suspended pending a psychological evaluation. At 12 years old I needed a psychologist to tell my school that it was safe for me to return. ED was so relieved that we had a break from school. I got to do what I wanted all day and didn't have to be near food. I didn't have to explain to people that I wasn't hungry or stand in the lunch line dreading them putting food on my tray. Suspension, though terrifying, was an ED dream. I liked giving ED what he wanted. It hurt when I didn't. The thoughts were all consuming and scary when I didn't, so I almost always did.

Not long after, I was cleared to go back to school they expelled me. They did not give a reason. All they told me was that they would always remember my smiling face running through the halls, but that I could no longer attend the school. My smiling face. I got suspended for hurting myself, but they would always remember my smiling face. I was a troubled child that didn't fit the mold of what they wanted, so I had to leave. They wouldn't even let me say goodbye to my friends. They took me up to my locker and when my friend approached me to ask why I was crying, the therapist told her, I didn't want to talk about it. I was showing that pain they were scared of; showing the emotions they didn't want me to have. There was too much pain behind my smiling face; there was too much turmoil following in my shadow. ED was no longer hiding in my shadow. ED had consumed me.

After spending a few weeks home to recover from the horror of being expelled, I transferred to public school. To say that this was a whole new world for me, would be an understatement. I had been in the same school with the same 60 kids since kindergarten and now I was at a new school with 300 kids in my grade. My first day of school, I witnessed a fight in the cafeteria and all I wanted to do was cry and go home. I got the hang of public school rather quickly though because of how I dressed and because of ED. There were other people like me who didn't eat lunch and who hurt themselves. People who wore black all the time and hid behind smiles and laughter. I actually felt like I fit in more there than I did at my old school. That is until I met my new demon.

I won't say his name, but my new demon wasn't one in my head. He wasn't one that only I could hear, but he was one that only I feared. My new demon used new tactics like telling me he loved me or telling me that I would be nothing without him. My new demon was just like ED, only everyone could see him. Everyone saw us together, after all… he was my boyfriend. I loved him. I would have done anything for him, and I did. I did everything for him and that made it easy to do everything for ED because nine times out of ten, they were in agreement. The biggest thing they agreed on was that I wasn't good enough. It took a long time for me to get away from that demon. It took a lot of traumatic experiences and lessons that I had to learn the hard way for him to finally set me free.

I didn't leave that demon. To be honest, I don't know if I would have had the strength to leave him as I have wondered during my relapses if I'll ever fully have the strength to let go of ED. When he set me free, I was terrified. I believed all the awful things he told me about myself. I believed I was nothing without him and I believed that well past middle school, high school and even into adulthood. Sometimes, even now in my late 20s, I catch myself wondering what I am worth and remembering his words.

I finished middle school with scrapes, bruises, and a broken-down soul. I was a tattered piece of person from what I once was and that is saying something since I wasn't much going into the relationship to begin with. I try and close my eyes sometimes really tight and remember back to the little blonde-haired, blue-eyed girl before ED, before the demons and remember a happier time. I look at home videos and hear my laugh and it makes me want to cry. Who is that girl? Did she know that all of this is ahead of her? I want to jump through the screen and put the precious little innocent girl in a bubble and protect her from all of the tears and razors and fists and words that were coming her way. I wished that I could protect her from ever creating this particular shadow… but, I am her… and I couldn't protect myself.

Memories of a Mother

Throughout Aly's years in middle school and high school, she had to struggle in so many ways. Many of her struggles resulted in self-esteem issues that left her vulnerable to the influence of others and to the strong voices of ED. Outwardly, most of the time, no one knew. I suspected but did nothing and for that, I will always feel a horrible measure of guilt. Unfortunately, I did not know enough about the disease and, although I sought help for her and took her to psychologists, they were not the right ones to help our daughter.

Several events occurred during middle school that, in my opinion, changed her life forever. When she started middle school, she also started cutting. I knew that cutting was a behavior that signified a need for control, that she felt the need to control something in her life and did so by cutting. When cutting, the person controls the depth of the cuts and the pain, providing a release of other pain that the individual is feeling. I wish that, back then, I would have associated Aly's desperate need for control with developing eating disorders. Sadly, I didn't.

Most people did not understand the cutting. I had "friends" approach me and tell me that my daughter was suicidal or suffering from mental illness. Seriously? These people had no idea about anything, especially, about why children cut. Some of these individuals didn't want their children playing with Aly. I could never understand why, since cutting is not contagious. It was Aly's personal way of gaining a measure of control. These days were just the beginning of darker days ahead and Aly's having to assert control over those things that caused her pain; control that she had by listening to the voice of ED.

In seventh grade, we were called to come to her private school for a meeting with the headmaster. Right away, we knew that was trouble. In the meeting, we were told that our daughter was being suspended immediately for allegedly having a knife in school and showing it to other students. Of course, no one could produce the knife but that didn't matter. She was suspended and told not to return until we had her evaluated by a psychologist who would state that it was safe for her to return. Unbelievable! No proof. No evidence. Just conjecture and her life and our family were turned upside down.

We did as we were told and took her to the psychologist. The psychologist found nothing wrong with her and sent the letter to the school advising that there was no reason Aly could not return. Thinking back on the encounter with the psychologist, I realize now what a fool he was. Our precious daughter was cutting regularly, struggling with an eating disorder, and inwardly, she was miserable. But the psychologist gave her a clean bill of health. Too bad it has been too many years to sue the bastard.

Aly returned to school, but her return was short-lived. The next notification was to come and pick her up because she had been expelled. I was in complete shock. They pulled her from class with no reason, had her collect her belongings, and go to the office. She was not allowed to say goodbye to her friends and was completely broken. If her emotional state had not been low before, this action sent her plummeting. She went to a dark place and, despite her smile, her eyes told a different story. Aly spent much of the next several years in that dark place spending more time listening to ED and not listening to anyone else. She also became a master of hiding her behaviors and pain from everyone in her life who loved her so much.

After the expulsion from the private school she had attended since kindergarten, Aly had to attend public school. She went from a school with several hundred students in grades K-8 to a school that had several hundred students in each grade. Her first day was so sad. After dropping her off, I cried all the way to work. She looked lost, surrounded by a sea of new faces, away from everything and everyone that she knew. Added to the emotional turmoil that she was dealing with, it is a wonder that she survived that day. But, survive she did. Unfortunately, she did so by listening to the ED voices in her head and later, listening to the destructive voice of her so-called boyfriend.

The story that I relate now was not known to any of us while it transpired. We learned about most of it when the father of the boy (who shall remain nameless) showed up at our home wanting to have our son arrested. He said that Greg had threatened his son, making it clear that Greg would kill this boy if he ever came near Aly again. We offered to call the police while he was there and explain what it was that his son did to our daughter that prompted the threat. He backed off after that.

There were some bright moments in the midst of the darkness. We celebrated Aly's bat mitzvah with a weekend of family meals, many friends including many from her old school, and a formal party to culminate the weekend's celebration. It was everything that she asked for and she was so happy that weekend. We actually saw some of the "old" Aly during that time. Unfortunately, those happy times were short-lived, and she quickly reverted to the "new" Aly, into that dark place where she found comfort and solace listening to ED.

Besides having hit her on more than one occasion and inflicting other means of physical pain, Aly's boyfriend emotionally tortured her. This boy convinced her that ED was right. She was fat and no one but this boy would ever love her. He began dictating to her what she could and could not eat, always reminding her that it was because he loved her that he would not let her eat what she wanted or eat at all. ED was in all its glory and Aly went further into the dark place, living life as a shadow of her true self.

By the time Aly finished middle school, it was hard to see the beautiful, happy little girl we all loved. She was so sad and even with anti-depressants, the sadness was ever present. Putting your child on anti-depressants before she is even a teenager is justification for parents to go on anti-depressants too. Because she had no fat on her body and was being seen by doctors who are not properly trained to treat depression in young girls and young girls with eating disorders, she was actually poisoned by the anti-depressants because the doctor increased the dosage. I will never forget the morning that she came into the living room, barely able to stand, in tears. "Mommy, I can't stand," she cried. "My legs are so weak, and everything tastes like metal." We quickly picked her up and carried her frail little body to the car. The emergency room physician told us that the anti-depressant had been building up in her bloodstream because she had no fat on her body and fat is usually where the chemical builds up to help the patient. The build-up in her bloodstream caused the metal taste and the severe weakness in her legs and arms. We had to wean her off of the medicine and find another doctor who, maybe, would not almost kill our child with the wrong dose of anti-depressants.

During those years, Aly regularly went to a therapist. Similar to other therapists that she had seen, her eating disorder was completely missed. Whether it was missed because she was/is a good actress or because of the physician's lack of training and knowledge is unknown. I suspect it was a combination of things. Whatever it was, Aly was not getting help. She was getting worse. There were times that the only way we could get her to eat was to tell her that, if she ate, she could visit her friend who was, at that time, in Shepard Pratt's Eating Disorder Unit. This was an in-patient facility for adolescents with eating disorders. Her friend was bulimic and, wouldn't you know, she taught Aly all about purging. God, how I wish I knew then... How I wish, I could turn the clock back and make other decisions along the way.

I think that, by now, you have an understanding of our Aly and what transpired up until she got to high school.

51

Chapter 3

Eating disorders do not discriminate. They affect people
from all religious, ethnic, and socioeconomic
backgrounds.[3]

He Didn't Stand in the Shadow.
He was the Shadow.

—   Alycia Oppenheim

Before beginning freshman year, we met with the student resource officer at the high school and the guidance counselor. We explained to them what had happened to me with my boyfriend the year before and everyone thought it best that we create my schedule to make sure I wouldn't bump into him in the halls. We all worked together in order to make me feel safe. The resource officer told me that if anything happened or if I felt unsafe to let him know and he would take care of it. I appreciated it, but ED and I knew how we would handle anything that happened. We were a team after all.

High school comes with pressures even if you aren't struggling with an eating disorder and other demons. There are cliques and for some, their bodies are still changing. You spend almost the whole freshman year trying to figure out where you fit. That is not how I spent my freshman year. I spent my freshman year dodging my ex and hiding within the confines of my thoughts. During my freshman year, my self-harming got very bad and my ex was going back and forth between trying to get me back and writing me notes to call me a "ho." I decided to write a book to help release my feelings. I also thought that maybe if I wrote what I went through and people read it, they would think twice before hurting themselves or it could help them leave a traumatic situation. I would sit in math assistance class and write (that is probably why I needed assistance in math). At the end, I had a short book entitled: Behind the Smile: Thoughts and Feelings of a Teenage Girl. I published it but didn't promote it. Writing the book didn't change the situation. Both demons were still lurking.

Part of the way through freshman year, I got so tired of feeling like I had to hurt myself that I told my parents that we either had to move away or I was dropping out of school. I couldn't handle being at that school anymore. I couldn't handle seeing the demon (who was my ex) anymore. I couldn't handle him hanging outside my classrooms or passing me notes through people. I didn't want to even be in the same state as him. ED fed off of this. The thoughts in my head were traumatizing and the words I was cutting into my legs were abusive. I needed a change.

My parents told me that if they found a house in Florida that we could move. I wanted to move. I wanted to stop being miserable, didn't I? When they returned from their trip to Florida and told us that they had found a house, I had so many emotions. I was excited at first because I thought it would be a fresh start, and I could let go of my demons. However, I was also terrified because ED made me believe that if we moved, I wouldn't be happy. He told me that I was incapable of being happy unless I had him. The excitement was gone because at least one demon was going to be following me. The shadow was forever there, and I was nothing without it.

The summer after my freshman year of high school, my family packed up the house and moved all of our worldly possessions to Fort Lauderdale, Florida. My family thought that it was just the four of us, but little did they know that a fifth was tagging a long and was getting more powerful as the days went on. No one knew what life in Florida would bring, but ED had some ideas.

Memories of a Mother

During Aly's years in middle school, my husband and I began talking about moving. Aly was all for it. She would welcome a new place, a place where nobody knew her history. A place that would be far away from the "boyfriend" and maybe, a place without the demons. The problem was that Greg was finishing high school and he did not want to move. He wanted to graduate with his friends, many of whom he had been in school with since kindergarten. What to do?

We talked about Jeff moving with Aly for a year and me staying behind in Baltimore with Greg. We could swap kids for weekends and holidays so that they would not miss us so much, and we would not miss them. This was not a viable option, for any of us. As it turned out, Aly was okay with staying in Baltimore one more year and starting high school there. It was decided. Greg would graduate with his friends and we would move somewhere in time for Aly to start her sophomore year.

Somewhere ended up being South Florida. Jeff and I found a house in Dania Beach. Our offer was accepted and suddenly, everything that we had been talking about for several years was imminent. I notified my employer that we were moving and thankfully, I was able to keep my job and would work virtual from that point forward. For me, the hard part came when I had to tell my dad we were moving. It worked out well for about seven years, until he got too sick to travel and then died in 2014. That is a different story entirely. Jeff gave notice to his employer, Greg and Aly said goodbye to their friends and in less than 90 days, the Oppenheim family was heading south. A new home in a new state. Would Aly's demons stay in Baltimore or would they cross the borders into Florida? Sadly, like all shadows, ED stayed close to her and came with us to Florida.

Chapter 4

Eating disorders have the highest mortality rate among mental illnesses.[4]

I moved to Florida after the traumatic experiences that helped develop my eating disorder. At 15, I was starting a new school with new people and I wasn't entirely sure what I was going to do with myself. I was leaving Baltimore for a reason. I needed a new start, but I didn't want a new start that would have me meeting new people. It would just be more people for me to compare myself to, more people to whom I would feel inferior.

As soon as I arrived at my new school, it felt like everything was crashing around me. The peer counselor assigned to show me around the school, didn't show up and I had no friends; I didn't know anyone. I was so alone, and I just wanted to go home. I just wanted to throw up or restrict, but all I could do was sit in the hallway and cry. Thankfully, the principal of the school was contacted by my mother and happened to be a wonderful woman. She helped get me settled on my first day. She took me around the school herself.

Everywhere I went, there was a new person for me to compare myself to and it was terrifying. I didn't have anyone to talk to about it either, which made it even harder. As time went on, I became more comfortable in one of my classrooms with my creative writing teacher. I began spending my lunch time in her classroom so that I didn't have to sit alone during lunch and look like the loser I felt I was. As the days and weeks went on, she started spending more of the lunch period in the room with me and getting to know me. She'd ask me questions about where I was from and about who I was. She seemed curious about me and I didn't mind because even though she was a teacher, she was the closest thing I had to a friend, outside of a few people that only spoke to me during class.

One day she brought up that she never really saw me eat. She began talking to me about eating disorders. The only thing I really knew about eating disorders, I knew from my friend who had been hospitalized and who had taught me about purging. When my friend got hospitalized for her eating disorder, I started using what she taught me about purging so that I could visit her in the hospital. I didn't think that I had a problem though. I didn't really think that what I was doing was abnormal. I just wasn't hungry, and I didn't like food. Weren't other "normal" people like that?

My teacher began telling me a story about a friend of hers that passed away from anorexia. I didn't understand why she was telling me this because in my head this couldn't happen to me. In my head, I wasn't sick. I just didn't like food. I could eat if I wanted to, I just didn't want to. I felt sorry that she had lost her friend, but I didn't relate to what her friend went through. At least, I didn't think that I related. Looking back now, I realize that I related and just didn't want to admit it because that would be admitting that I had a problem. If I did that, then I would have to give up what I thought was my best friend, my shadow and something I thought was my safety blanket. I thanked my teacher for telling me the story but explained that I didn't have an eating disorder. I even lied and told her that I did eat my meals, and I didn't know what she was talking about. ED was proud of the lie.

After that, when I did eat lunch in her classroom, I made sure that other people were in the room with me so that she could concentrate on other people and not pay attention to my lack of intake. Over time, I did make friends, but they didn't notice or make it known to me that they noticed that I didn't eat at lunch time. We would laugh, and people watch while we stood in the corner. It made me feel better that I had friends and people to talk to, but I did not dare talk about food or about eating disorders because in my mind, I still did not have one. It was not until junior year when I was dating this one guy that I even said the words, "I have an eating disorder." Even then, I did nothing about it. He didn't know that we were supposed to do anything about it, so he didn't tell my parents and I never told them either.

I once voiced to my therapist that I thought that I might have a problem. She had done her dissertation and master's concentration on eating disorders, so I thought, she would be the one to ask if I had one. She told me I had disordered eating, but not an eating disorder. I took this to mean that nothing was wrong with me and I could go on doing as I was doing, and it wouldn't matter. This means that what I was doing was normal and not wrong, right?

Memories of a Mother

The summer of 2005 was filled with so many goodbyes and very few reasons for me to be happy. We were fleeing the place that I had called home for all but three years of my entire life. I was leaving my office, friends, and home, traveling to parts unknown. I was also leaving my dad, who had been my security and confidant about so much. There were a few positives about moving to Florida. My favorite aunt was there (she died not long after we moved); my niece, her husband, and adorable baby girl (they moved to Baltimore a short time after we moved to Florida and then divorced); my mom; and youngest brother. Unfortunately, none of those positives outweighed the feelings I had as we left on the auto-train and I waved goodbye to my dad. We were on our way. Jeff, Greg, Aly, and ED, her ever-present shadow.

Aly's first day of school got off to a terrible start. Within twenty minutes of the school day beginning, Aly called me from her cell phone in tears, almost hysterical. She was alone in the hallway, the person who was supposed to show her around did not show, and she was lost. My heart was breaking. I told her to calm down and that I would call school. Little did I know that the storm we had the night before took out the phone lines and I could not reach anyone. I finally reached the school district who contacted the principal. She called me from her cell phone, and I explained what was happening and described where Aly said she was sitting. I will forever be grateful to this woman who let me cry my heart out on the phone and then went to help my daughter.

Aly seemed to have made a few friends in high school. One very special friend, we affectionately called, "The Voice." He would call every evening to let her know that he would pick her up for school the next day. I did not meet the person behind "The Voice" for a long time, but he took her to school almost every day. Aly remains best friends with this boy (now a married man with a beautiful new daughter) and I will always be grateful to him for all that he has done for her. (I am certain that he does not even realize the positive influence and effect he has had on her life for so many years.)

Life went on and Aly seemed, on the surface, to be adjusting. She loved her creative writing teacher and even submitted a poem to the Broward County Lit Fair. She won second place and was published in the school's Lit Magazine. Even then, she was so talented and was able to express herself beautifully in writing and yet, could not express her feelings to me, her father, or her brother. She could not articulate the pain that she was in or that she lived with a shadow that engulfed her all of the time. I picture ED as a Death Eater from Harry Potter. Always looming over top of her, a big shadow that consumes a part of her soul.

Chapter 5

Turn, Pivot and Smile, it will
drive ED nuts.

— *Alycia Oppenheim*

When I was 16, I received a call from a place called Barbizon. Someone had nominated me to go to an audition for modeling school. I didn't know who and I didn't fully understand why they had chosen me, but I had been chosen. I was terrified. I was shy and contained within myself. The thought of talking to people, going into a room, and "showing them what I've got," made me shake and feel sick. Little did anyone know though, I really wanted to be a model. I wanted to be in fashion shows and walk the runway. I was far too short to do so, but it was a kind of dream of mine to have that kind of confidence, to not fear falling on my face, and look beautiful in the pictures. I didn't think I deserved the nomination or the interview, but I talked it over with my boyfriend. He thought it was a great idea and thought I completely deserved it. He thought, I'd be crazy not to at least go to the audition. My mom agreed. So, with my mom and my boyfriend in tow, we drove down the street to the audition.

I don't know what came over me while I was there, but I spun, and smiled, and I did what was asked. I killed that audition and they asked me to be a part of that term of their school. I was a student of Barbizon and I had no idea at the time what that meant.

Barbizon was truly an incredible experience for me, and I thank them for all of the tools they gave me, tools that I continue to use every day. They gave me the confidence that I lacked and helped me find the courage to speak up and to speak out. I learned to publicly speak at Barbizon and without that tool, I would not have achieved much of what I did. Without the confidence and courage, I would not have won the awards that I did. I would not have been able to help the countless number of women and girls I had helped through my time as an AmeriCorps member with Women in Distress of Broward County. Barbizon taught me to try and to believe in myself. They also taught me etiquette and how to apply make-up (and how to make a music video).

ED hated my time at Barbizon because, during those days, I was able to ignore him. I mean, I didn't really eat when we were supposed to, but I didn't listen to him when he told me to compare myself to the other girls. I didn't listen to him or hold his hand when I had to do something scary. I let the teachers be my guides because after all, that is what they were there for. ED wanted me to quit so badly. He wanted me to camp out in my room and be shy or camp out in my boyfriend's room and let him ignore me. ED wanted my unhealthy behaviors and not the ones that Barbizon was teaching me. Barbizon gave me an escape that I hadn't had except for with Shakespeare, and it helped create the healthy parts of me. Barbizon hid my shadow even if for just a few hours on two Saturdays a month.

Memories of a Mother

When Aly came home and told us about the offer to audition for Barbizon, we were shocked. We had heard of Barbizon but had never thought about sending Aly. Now she had the opportunity to audition for Barbizon. Her emotions went from anxiety to excitement, from fear to anticipation. I know that she had always wanted to be a model and, while runway modeling was not an option (Aly is only 5' tall), there might be other opportunities. Certainly, just the experience of auditioning for Barbizon and getting accepted would boost her self-esteem and it could be fun.

We went to the audition and Aly performed so well. She exuded such confidence and poise, neither of which did she possess in abundance. Before leaving the audition, she was invited to start in the next Barbizon class. We left the hotel and for that short time, my little girl with the bright blue, happy eyes was beaming and there were no shadows.

The Barbizon experience was one of the best experiences of Aly's life. They taught her so much about make-up, how to dress, how to carry herself, how to speak, and project her voice. They instilled a confidence in her and inspired her to go outside of her comfort zone. These lessons have remained with her ever since and I credit Barbizon with having made a monumental difference in Aly's life. After Barbizon, Aly was willing to stand up in front of a room full of people and speak. She was not afraid to talk to groups of any size about topics ranging from teen awareness about HIV and AIDs to domestic violence, bullying, and self-harming. Barbizon helped shatter the shell that surrounded her, and for this, I shall always be grateful to them and to the unknown person who gave Barbizon, Aly's name.

Chapter 6

The rest of high school went by as a blur. I made a lot of decisions that I am not proud of and decisions that hurt people that I cared about. I would want to blame ED for these decisions. Blame ED for wanting attention from other people so much that I hurt the person that was there for me the most. I finished high school with a high GPA and won awards for my service to the community and public speaking. As I grew up, my decisions in my personal life began becoming more vicious. I once made the man I was seeing go on a week-long search for ipecac for me because I wanted a new way to purge. I manipulated my way into making him do something that he knew would hurt me, but he did it anyway because he loved me.

ED convinced me that these were things that I needed, attention and new ways to adhere to ED's rules. I thought that as long as I had my symptoms and I had my eating disorder, everything was going to be okay. I had this numb feeling deep within me that made me almost heartless. I loved my boyfriend at the time. I built a life around him. But the numbness that I felt and the symptoms that I needed to use, made it hard for me to devote myself to him or anyone. I still struggle with this.

I decided I needed to change and make something more of myself. I wanted to have at least a part of me of which I could be proud. I started college with a full-time job, working as an AmeriCorps member and youth prevention educator at a domestic violence agency as well as going to school full-time. I may not have been proud of who I was on the outside, but I was beginning to be proud of who I was on the inside.

Unfortunately, even with all of my accomplishments, ED was still around. I won awards, received great evaluations and yet I still wasn't eating. Life was also difficult because I was just learning to live on my own, so I didn't have anyone watching me and telling me to eat. It was time to grow up and be an adult. ED decided that even as an adult eating was not an option. ED still controlled most of my life. I finished my AA with a high GPA and finished my AmeriCorps service. It was time to move on to my bachelor's degree, but even as I moved to Tampa, ED was still there, still lurking in the shadows.

Memories of a Mother

With all of the bad times, the tears, the pain, and hurt, there were good days and bright times along the way. By the end of 10th grade, Aly had become recognized as THE peer counselor. Whenever difficult situations arose, it was Aly who was called upon to help her peers. This recognition permitted her to be the only senior with permission to have her cell phone on throughout the day.

When Aly started high school in Florida, we learned about the Silver Knights program. This program recognizes outstanding students who maintain good grades and who apply their knowledge and/or talents to contribute to their communities. Most students who try for a Silver Knights award start working on their projects in middle school. Aly was going into 11th grade and time was short, but Aly decided she wanted to win Silver Knights and so the endeavor began.

Suffice to say that Aly did not win Silver Knights that year, but she did win Silver Knights Honorable Mention for her project – the first (ever) teens march for HIV and AIDS awareness. The mayor of Hollywood presented her with a proclamation, and she received proclamations from the governor and President Bush. Over 100 students and young adults marched the length of the Hollywood Beach Broadwalk to bring awareness to HIV and AIDS. It was an incredible day and an amazing project. Truth be told, if her project had not been so controversial, we all believe she would have come in first.

During her senior year, Aly's accomplishments also earned recognition from other areas. The Hollywood Jaycees named her the Outstanding High School Student of Hollywood, Florida and the Florida Jaycees honored her as the Outstanding Young Floridian. The entire family attended the dinner in Daytona when the honorees received their awards. It was an incredible evening and a culmination to a very successful school year. For a period of time, ED was well into the shadows and Aly was able to enjoy her accomplishments. Sadly, ED would not leave her alone and the time was coming when ED would move from the shadows and consumer her spirit.

Chapter 7

I drank the cold liquid as it shot into my core.
I was looking for answers, but all
I found was ED.

—   Alycia Oppenheim

I spent a considerable amount of time wondering if I had an eating disorder before ever getting help. Even after my therapist told me I didn't have an eating disorder, my teacher's' words resonated with me, and I still questioned whether I had one or not. The first time I really admitted that I had an eating disorder was when I was 17, and I was confiding in my boyfriend how I felt about myself. I told my boyfriend that I thought I was fat and disgusting and that I didn't eat. I said that I didn't like myself and that I had an eating disorder. He didn't know what that meant. I don't think that either of us really knew what that meant. Even after that confession, I still didn't get help until I was 20. By then, I had destroyed my body so much that I was quickly speeding toward an outcome of which there was no turning back. I was killing myself and if I didn't do something soon, I would have succeeded.

When I was living in Tampa for school, my purging got worse. There was a time where I was bleeding and the pain was excruciating, but ED was so far in control that I couldn't stop the behaviors. I was in and out of hospitals for weeks, trying to figure out what was causing the stomach and chest pains, but no doctors had any answers for me. I went to four hospitals. I had so many doctors pump me with drugs but never give me any answers. I went to one hospital that tried to send me home before giving me medications or tests.

I finally went to see a gastroenterologist, and he did an endoscopy. The endoscopy showed that I had gastritis and esophagitis. I had a partial hole through my esophagus and acid eroding my stomach. My stomach was basically black from the acid. The pictures were disgusting. He told me that if I kept purging and kept the lifestyle that I was living, I may not make it another three years. This news was shocking. I squeezed my mother's hand as I heard the news, but it didn't feel like her hand squeezing me back. It was ED's. All he heard was, "no more purging, no more restricting." I knew it was time to get help.

My first treatment was an intensive outpatient facility in Tampa. I went to group a few days a week and spoke with women and girls that understood where I was coming from. It was the first time I could relate to people. Unfortunately, part of this program was having to have meals with these people. I didn't like that part. I didn't last long going to IOP. I continued going to groups every so often and was also attending AA meetings. Unfortunately, I didn't like the people running the eating disorder facility so it was best for me to just leave.

My trips to AA weren't necessarily because I had an addiction to drinking. I drank to further my eating disorder and because of that my drinking got out of control. It was easier for me to say I had a drinking problem than to admit that my eating disorder was out of control. People understood alcoholism and didn't think alcoholism made you crazy. People didn't say, "Why don't you just stop drinking?" like they said, "why don't you just eat?" I figured that if I got help for one problem, maybe that would help the other. It got to the point where I had bottles of alcohol all around my room. Some were mixed with Gatorade; others were just regular bottles. There was beer and vodka mostly. A few times a week, I had Mike's Hard Lemonade or wine coolers.

I made a really bad decision while drunk one night and when I woke up the next morning, I changed my phone number and poured all the alcohol down the sink. Sometimes, when I am feeling low and I let ED take control, I let other demons in, and that is what I did the night before I gave up drinking. I contacted my biggest demon besides ED, and I told him things. I agreed to things that I should never and would never have if I had been sober. Alcohol had changed me; ED and alcohol together had changed me. That night after I threw out all of the alcohol, I went to my first AA meeting.

I had a sponsor, but she dropped me because she said that I didn't take the steps seriously. The problem was that I was taking them seriously. I was trying to work the steps, but working steps based on a belief in a higher power is difficult when you struggle with a belief in God. She felt I was mocking her when I told her that William Shakespeare was my higher power. I wasn't mocking her. When I was going through my traumatic experiences when I was a young teen, it was the writings of Shakespeare that got me through. If I was stuck in a basement with nothing to do, or stuck in the deep corners of my mind, it was Shakespeare's words that helped me escape the turmoil, and it was

Shakespeare's canon that gave me a safe place to be when the whole world felt like a never-ending field of land mines. Shakespeare was and is my higher power and she just didn't understand that. My time in AA didn't last very long, but the drinking stopped.

I spent my time in Tampa working through ED, alcohol and what I now learned was my bipolar disorder. I made decisions for weeks that were not thought out and some that were unsafe. I would then crash into a whirlwind of debilitating depression. I don't know how I made it through school and earned my bachelor's degree.

I wasn't diagnosed with bipolar disorder until late in my 20s. Looking back at those dark days, I can see so many times when I wish that I had been on my medication so that situations wouldn't have happened or would have been better controlled. I wonder how much of my shadow I could have left at home instead of brought to school had I been properly medicated while in university. But alas, my shadow followed me to classes on my mile walk through campus. He held my hand as I crossed the road, trying to decide if I was going to stop and get that bagel before class. Nine times out of ten, I didn't stop.

Luckily, I had a good friend at school that liked to fight with ED. She would cook me dinner and make me laugh and smile. She would help me pick the foods I liked and when ED would take control and tell me not to eat, she would tell me, I couldn't come over if I wasn't going to eat. She knew I hated to be alone and that would help force me to eat at least a small amount. Without her, I don't know if I would have finished my final year of school. I am forever grateful for her and her strength in my battle against ED.

Memories of a Mother

After high school, Aly attended Broward College and worked for Women in Distress (WID) of Broward County as an AmeriCorps member. From an introverted child, she had blossomed into an amazing public speaker. She was able to channel the terrible events of middle school into her speaking and quickly became THE speaker for many meetings throughout the tri-county area. She also excelled teaching students from kindergarten through 12th grade about various topics from bullying to date rape and many subjects in between.

Broward College and working for WID were excellent experiences for Aly. Although, at the time we did not know the extent of her problems, ED remained ever-present in her life, along with depression and other demons. In school and while teaching or speaking, the dark shadow of ED that was always with her, seemed to have lightened just a bit. She was doing well, was highly regarded by her peers and bosses and graduated with her AA in two years.

With her AA degree, Aly set her sights on the bachelor's degree and was accepted at University of South Florida in Tampa. As luck would have it, a good friend and co-worker lived in Tampa and her mother lived alone in a two-

bedroom apartment. Aly, being able to live there would be a win-win for both of them. She had a beautiful room in a great development not far from school, and a landlady who was phenomenal. The fact that Jan was also a nurse would quickly elevate her from landlady to life-saver and a dear friend forever.

Not long after moving to Tampa, Aly began having stomach aches. At first, when we spoke about it, she downplayed the discomfort but all that changed over time. Aly ended up visiting the emergency rooms at several different hospitals because of the severity of her pain. The third or fourth time (I can't remember which), I was finally told what was happening. Suffice to say, we were terrified as we had no idea what could possibly be wrong. (At this point, we had no idea the extent of her eating disorder.) The hospital advised her to see a gastroenterologist and, thankfully, Jan had worked for one of the best and set her up with the practice.

The GI doctor ordered an endoscopy, so I drove up to Tampa the night before and took her for the procedure. There are no words to describe the anguish, anxiety, and fear that struck at the very core of my being when he showed both Aly and me the pictures of her esophagus and stomach. Her purging and restrictive behaviors were causing the acids in her stomach to literally burn a hole in her esophagus and damage her stomach. The GI doctor was very clear when he told her that continuing those behaviors would kill her. Not could. Would. My precious daughter, the beautiful baby girl that I brought into this world was slowly killing herself because of the voice of ED.

That day, the truth about everything came tumbling out. We spoke for hours. We cried together. We hugged a lot and we planned. Aly did not want to die and did not want to keep living in pain. I was filled with guilt, fear, pain, and anguish; did not know where to turn or what to do. It was Aly herself who provided the answers. She made it clear that her dealing with ED was not my fault; her being sick was her doing and she, alone, had to stop listening to ED, had to eat, and get healthy.

Before leaving Tampa, Aly and I went to see an intensive outpatient treatment (IOP) center in Tampa. Aly agreed to go, and Jan offered to help monitor her to be sure that she was taking the prescribed medicines and eating her meals. I returned home with a heavy heart, my mind racing and imagining the worse; afraid to close my eyes because of the nightmares that were sure to come.

IOP did not last very long. Aly tried some other programs, including AA but nothing seemed to be the right fit. At the end of the term, despite her being given a clean bill of health from the GI doctor for the gastritis and esophagitis, it was decided that Aly should take a medical leave of absence and return home. We packed up her belongings, said a tearful goodbye to Jan, and headed home with our daughter and the dark shadow, we now all knew as ED.

Chapter 8

"As someone supporting someone with an cating disorder,
I constantly felt like I'd lost; like I didn't know how I
could help you."

— Greg Oppenheim (brother)

***I feared walking in the doors in the beginning
and I feared walking out the doors at the end.***

*— **Alycia Oppenheim***

It was a year or so after that when I decided that I should seek out more help. It took a lot to make the decision to go to residential treatment. I made pros and cons lists, I discussed it with my family; I discussed it with my boyfriend at the time. Part of me didn't feel like I needed it, and then the more logical side of me knew that I was in serious trouble if I didn't take the help that was being offered to me. I think the biggest fear for me in going to residential treatment was that I would have to try for recovery, and similar to the other times I had tried outpatient treatment, I wasn't sure that recovery was what I wanted. Recovery meant that I was giving up something that was a part of who I was; I felt that my identity was made up of my eating disorder. I was the sick girl. If I was going to give up ED, I would no longer have an identity and the unknown was terrifying.

After discussing in great detail all of my options and the best route to take, we all decided that it was best for me to go to residential treatment. I still didn't want to go, and I was petrified to leave my life in New York and my boyfriend; to leave what I knew. I remember looking in the mirror the day before my mom arrived to take me to Philadelphia for treatment and with all the negative thoughts that were rushing through my brain like a train there was one that stuck out. The thought was that no matter where I go and no matter how hard I try, I would never be free from ED and I would never like myself. I had spent so many years with ED. He followed me to Florida when I was a child. He followed me to Tampa when I went to college and New York after that. What if I could never be without ED? What if it was impossible? These thoughts that ran shivers through me almost made me just tell everyone to forget it; I would just stay and spend however long ED would give me with the people I loved. However, I pushed through and I packed my stuff, said goodbye to my boyfriend and I hopped on a bus to Philadelphia where I would meet my mom and go to my first and only residential treatment center.

I tried to think of other things and happy things on the way there so that my fear and anxiousness didn't take over. It didn't work very well. One of my biggest fears, besides that of letting go of my identity, was that I wasn't going to get along with any of the girls. I thought they would be skinnier than me and prettier than me and it would just be like every other time I see females. I would just end up comparing myself to them. Even before I got there and met anyone it seemed like a competition; something that is very prevalent in eating disorder treatment centers.

The disease makes you want to believe that you aren't sick enough so that much of the time when people with eating disorders are staying in treatment centers, it becomes a competition to feel like you belong there. If the girls are skinnier or sicker than you, the eating disorder makes you believe that you don't belong there, and you failed at doing what you were told. The competition and perfectionism make it really hard to function the first few days or weeks being in residential treatment.

When I arrived, I sat in the main house with another girl that was entering treatment that day. She was thin and adorable; she had a peg tube in her nose. My ED shouted at me that this girl had what it took to be beautiful; I sat quietly as my mom talked with her parents. I felt like I was a little child waiting in the principal's office instead of a 21-year-old woman, trying to save her own life. I sat and listened. I went where I was told and answered questions like I was on autopilot. When it was time for lunch and time for my mom to leave, I began to cry. Why was I there? Why did they tell me I had to be there? I couldn't have been sick enough to be there. I didn't want my mom to leave. I didn't want to stay. It felt like the first day of preschool when your parents leave you with these strangers and you feel like you are being deserted and they don't love you anymore. But she left, and I stayed. A part of me felt like I was all alone in the world.

When the therapist brought me into lunch, she explained to me how trays worked. I was given a tray with all the food I was supposed to eat already on the tray. I was expected to eat everything. Sundays would be the day that we would choose what food we would have on our trays. If I did not eat it all, I would be supplemented with an Ensure drink. It being my first day and my first meal, I didn't eat. I cried through the whole meal and felt like I had made a huge mistake. I just wanted to go home, curl up with my boyfriend and forget about treatment or ED or life. It was not that easy, and I had to deal with that and learn to put my life together. I could have signed myself out as I was an adult, but my fear of disappointing everyone else overpowered my fear of being inside the facility.

As time went on, life in residential got easier. I made friends, enjoyed my groups, learned to knit, and crochet. I learned new games to play at meals that made getting through them easier. I remember spending everyday either watching Glee or watching Tangled with the girls, all of us knitting or crocheting something. It was peaceful and turned out to be an escape from everything in the world. On the weekends, I'd get visitors. My first weekend there my brother, two of my friends, and my boyfriend came to visit. We sat on the deck and played cards ignoring the fact that they were visiting me at a residential treatment center and I couldn't leave with them. They gave me laughs and attention, but when they left, it was even harder because I didn't want them to go. I was able to dismiss the sad feelings by going to my groups and spending time with my new friends, but when it was time for sleep and I laid in my bed with my roommate asleep in the bed next to mine, I missed my bed and my tiny New York apartment. I missed my life. I cried myself to sleep that night as the sleep medicine drifted into my system.

While I was in residential, my boyfriend asked permission from my brother to officially be with me and it made me sad that I was sitting in a treatment center instead of enjoying my new, official relationship. I feel like a lot of the time, I was looking for reasons not to be there; ways to leave, but at the end of the day, I was still there. I was still fighting the demons in my head and in my heart. It was still my choice to stay or go and despite all of the feelings, I stayed.

My therapist in treatment was great and very understanding, but it was hard for me to open up to another therapist and tell her all my secrets. Slowly, she broke down my walls and I confided in her all of my trauma and thoughts; the feelings I was still trying to come to terms with that I hadn't told anyone other than my boyfriend. I started to enjoy being there.

Residential became a sequence of days just running into one another. I went to groups, I ate my meals or got supplemented, went to more groups, went to doctors' appointments, and moved up the levels. As time went on, I was able to go out on leave either with other girls on my level or with my boyfriend when he came to visit. I lived in the residential bubble where nothing could hurt me. It was life with no drama. The treatment center was an escape from life. The only problem with this was that I was not prepared to leave. Most days, I didn't even think of leaving. I lived in this imaginary world where I could spend my days in treatment, knit, and have no problems. But at night, when it was time to go to sleep, I wanted to be in my bed with my boyfriend. I dreamt of a world that was not possible and yet that is what I thought of every day. I wanted parts of both worlds; the lack of drama from one world and the love from the other.

As time went on, the fear of leaving started to sink in. I got used to spending every day in my sweatpants, never having to put on real clothes, and the hardest decision, I needed to face, was on Sundays when we filled in our meal cards. Once I switched up to FO (Fix Own) and got to decide my own meals at mealtimes, I no longer had hard decisions. Life was so easy and repetitive in residential and I felt so safe. The outside world was becoming more and more distant. Even though I spoke to my family and my boyfriend every day, I couldn't imagine going back to the outside world and even more, I could not imagine going back to the outside world and being ED free. There were times when I was in residential that I didn't even think of my ED. It began feeling like sleepaway camp and I was just spending time with my friends and learning new things. Nothing about being there was scary anymore.

The only time that I would think of why I was there was in therapy. Therapy had me thinking about how this all started. With all of the therapists I had before, we never could pinpoint when ED first started or how. She couldn't figure out how, but we narrowed down a bit more of when it started with my mom's help during phone sessions.

We realized that I started self-harming after my eating disorder became the voice in my head. It's a memory I can't fully remember but can imagine. I remember a room and the blood dripping off my wrist, the sound of my stomach rumbling, still not used to the hunger pains. I imagine the voice behind it all. The voice saying that it was okay, that there was no other way. I was a young girl, around age ten and one day there was a voice that began speaking every time I ate. The voice spoke every time I cried. I would wake up some nights gasping for air and the voice would be there with its soothing tone telling me everything would be okay. I needed that voice. I needed to believe the beautiful words that it was telling me. I sat in that room, that dark room and watched the blood. I listened to the voice. I cut again.

My life wasn't very different than any other little girl's life, which probably is what made it so hard to pinpoint why it all happened. I went to school just like every other ten or eleven-year-old. I did my homework, I played with friends. I had crushes on boys in my school and giggled when they would pass me in the halls. On the outside, I was no different. My blonde hair and blue eyes weren't different. I wasn't tall or super short. I was just plain and ordinary. I was nothing special, no matter how hard I tried to be. I would flirt with the boys in my grade or above. I would manipulate them in hopes that if they gave me some attention, the voice in my head would stop. I made mistakes and I did stupid things in order to get that voice out of my head. I guess, looking back on it now, the things I tried didn't work because I didn't really want the voice to go away. Even now at age 29, and at 21 when I was in residential treatment and trying to figure out how this all happened to me, that voice was and is still with me. His name is ED. He has been my greatest ally and my worst enemy all in one for many years now and yet I still can't imagine my life without his voice. ED is the voice from when I was a little girl. He is like that creepy dolly that you've had since you were little that you know you should throw away but don't because of what it symbolizes. ED is my dolly. My demonic, evil dolly that tells me the truth, I think I need to hear; the truth, I believe to be fact no matter how many times I'm told it's false. The more time that I spent with my therapist, the more he came out and tried to battle the words she was saying.

Going through all this in my mind and discussing it with my therapist, I remembered wishing I had more attention. I imagined a little girl feeling alone while sitting at a table with the people she thought were her friends. I remembered fighting with my friends a lot. I remembered feeling betrayed and feeling that I was so different, but not different at all. I imagined the daydreams that I had sitting in class not being able to focus. I remembered thinking of the voice and wondering what it would say next. I remembered feeling like all the other girls were so much prettier than me; a feeling that was not much different than how I felt around the girls I was in treatment with. They were taller than me because, whereas I was not super short, I was still short. I remembered the boys giving them more attention and not understanding what was wrong with me. I remembered the voice explaining to me what was wrong. The voice said that there was something different about me and that difference was my body. It was okay though because the voice also came with a solution. If I stopped eating and I lost weight, the boys would like me. If I stopped eating, then the pain I was feeling would go away. I wanted the pain to go away even if I didn't know what was really causing the pain.

Cutting was an outlet for the pain as well. Feeling the pain of the cut, watching the blood, and hearing the voice made me believe that the pain was going away. I was still cutting when I went into treatment. They took my razors away and I had to ask permission for my razors once a week so that I could shave. I hated this. It made me feel like a child. I hated asking permission for things when I was older than half of the girls I was in treatment with, but I understood that because of my behavior the punishment was warranted. I guess.

The only problem when I was younger was that the more that I cut myself, the more that I stopped eating, the more I stopped caring. I learned over time to numb myself. I don't think that it made anyone like me more. I don't believe that I stopped getting bullied by the other girls or that my friends and I stopped fighting. None of it made me different in the ways I wanted to be. I wasn't mysterious or beautiful. I just couldn't feel the agonizing pain that I was feeling before. The haze over my life was still there. The voice was wrong. It was at this point that I learned not to argue with the voice. I learned that the voice cared about me and was the only one that cared about me.

I remember one day when the numbing began influencing my life. I was sitting in the computer room of my house and I had cuts on my arm. I don't remember why I was fighting with my parents, honestly at the time I was so numb, I probably didn't care, and my mom came in to yell at me. She didn't understand why I kept hurting myself. I remember her beginning to cry and she slid down the wall and began hitting her head on the wall. I don't remember what she was saying. My dad came in and tried to get her up and he began saying something to me as well, but the numbness tuned them out. I just stared at them. I felt nothing. ED made me feel nothing. I wish I could say that it hurt me. It hurts me now thinking back on the pain I caused them, but back then the numbness that the cutting and the eating disorder caused, I couldn't feel. ED was in control and it was terrifying if I didn't listen to him. I cared more about that than anything.

Through our talks, the therapist had me remembering the first time the voice yelled at me; yelled as if all it wanted was for me to hear it clearly. It yelled as if it just wanted to get through the haze that wasn't just over my eyes but transferred to white noise in my ears. There were times even ED couldn't break through the numbness. I needed to hear the words that it was saying and yet without yelling it couldn't break through. By the time I heard what the voice was saying it was all I could hear. Every other sound of the world was gone and all I heard was this voice. The voice told me that I was disgusting; that this was fact. The voice said, I was fat; that this was fact. The voice told me that I was annoying and obnoxious and that no one really liked me and that this too was fact. The voice told me that it wasn't wrong; I was just failing at listening and doing what I was told like I failed at doing everything else.

At the time, I was only skipping breakfast. The voice said that to really make changes, I had to skip lunch too. I had to lie and pretend that I wasn't but that if I didn't eat all day things would be different. I would be different. I believed this voice. I needed the voice. I trusted my dolly. I stopped eating. Unfortunately, it started at 10 and when I went to treatment at 21, the voice hadn't changed its tune and I felt like my dolly was still right. My therapist was trying to break through a decade of bad thoughts and self-hatred and sadly, before she truly got through, I left treatment.

Part of my mom's conditions with the treatment center was that they didn't tell me how much it was costing. My personality would put the money that it cost for treatment before my own health and knowing that, my mom told them not to speak to me about it. Unfortunately, there was one person who did not listen and as soon as she told me I began lying to my doctors. Thanks to my eating disorder, I was a master manipulator and I manipulated the system so that I could leave treatment with still "finishing the levels."

There are steps you have to take after leaving treatment and the next step was supposed to be day treatment. It is the easiest way to step down from 24-hour care. I convinced my team and the treatment center that I was going to go to IOP (intensive outpatient treatment) instead of day and that I would be okay. The team allowed it to happen and a week from the time I was told about the cost, my mom drove back up the driveway of the treatment center and this time I was right beside her. With my stomach and heart in my throat, I was sent back into the real world, completely terrified with the voice in my head telling me everything would be okay. Within days of being back home, I started using symptoms again.

Memories of a Mother

I remember answering my phone the day Aly decided she needed to be in residential treatment. My heart stopped, the tears came, but I found the strength to tell her it would be okay and that I would be there for her. I called my boss, booked my flight and the next day, I flew to Philadelphia. I remember sitting in the cab heading to the train station where Aly's Mega Bus would arrive. I could not stop crying, could not hold back the emotions. I was in a strange city, going to pick up my precious child and take her to a residential treatment center. How could things have gotten this bad? I was filled with guilt, self-loathing, and fear. Could they help penetrate the demons Aly was fighting? Could anyone?

That night, we went to dinner and had a great evening together. Although she was clearly frightened, she was resolute in her decision. She knew that she needed help and knew that residential was the only way. The next morning, we went together, hand-in-hand, through the doors of the place that would be her home for as long as it took.

When we arrived, Aly was taken by a staff person to her room, while I met with the administrator and signed papers and agreed to a payment plan that would have me writing checks every month for years but none of it mattered. All that mattered was that my daughter would get the help she so desperately needed. After signing the papers, I remember sitting in the family room, an area that looked like someone's living room. There was another family there, the parents and a young girl who looked to be eight or nine (she was actually 14). This child had a peg tube and was even worse off than Aly.

Aly and I were re-united, and she told me how her bags were searched. Everything was contraband. No phones were allowed. No sweet 'n low. No computers. She would have no contact with the outside world, but she would be permitted to call from a payphone each day.

The time came for me to leave. By then, Aly had met a few of the girls, each one fighting her own demons. We walked down the beautiful path together and God, how hard I tried to not let her see the devastation that I was feeling. I was about to get into a cab and ride off, leaving her at that place because I had failed her and could not help. I looked back, and she looked so helpless; so lost. This was her decision and it was the right decision. That didn't change the way that I felt or the look on her face that will haunt my dreams until I die.

Chapter 9

I'm at a crossroads with a blindfold on.
All I have are the voices in my head telling me which way
to go.
I hear a loud, thunderous voice telling me to go one way
for happiness.
It tells me to go its way to find what I seek and all the love
and attention I could want.
Quietly in the background, I hear a small sound telling me
to go the other way.
This almost whisper as if brushing by my ear like the wind
telling me down its path, I'll find what I deserve.

I'm at a crossroads with a blindfold on, but I know which
voice which is.
I know ED's voice tempting me with the body I want and
the love he thinks it'll win me.
ED tells me of a man who won't reject me and the
happiness I'll find in finally liking myself.
I know ED says beautiful words, but I know that he lies.

I'm at a crossroads, but I take the blindfold off.
I see ED standing on his path beckoning me to follow him.
There are just leaves blowing down the path of recovery;

A slight vision of something or someone that hasn't been formed yet.

I stand looking at my crossroads with the demon on one side and a silent whisper on the other.

I know which is easy and which is hard.

I sit at my crossroads and stare into two possible futures and wonder…

Will there ever stop being crossroads?

__Home is where you should be most happy...__
__but where is home?__

__—   Alycia Oppenheim__

I've never been one to easily find a place that feels like home. I have a home where my family is, but where I grew up in Baltimore, Florida or even New York never felt like home. I don't know if it is because I constantly feel like I don't fit in, but nowhere has ever felt like home to me. I look back at my time in Baltimore and even when I go and visit, it never feels like home, even though I was born there. I try and look within myself and even there does not feel like home. I am a stranger to myself at times. It could be that because of my eating disorder and it not allowing me to live within myself that I have never given a place an opportunity to feel like home. Everything is harder when you don't feel like you have a home; where you don't feel like you belong.

When I returned to New York after my time in Renfrew, life was much harder than I thought it was going to be. Within days of returning, I relapsed and was hearing the same voice that was in my head before I left. I had learned a few coping mechanisms, but it didn't help the way that I thought it would. Everyone in my life was supportive and was trying to help me get through the transition from residential to intensive outpatient (IOP), but within myself, it just didn't seem possible. When you leave residential treatment, the next logical step is to step down to Day treatment. I did not do that because I knew that would cost more money and I was not going to put my family through that. I was not going to be more of a burden. I spent so much time feeling like a burden. I felt like being born was a burden. My family had spent so much time and energy taking care of me, worrying about me, spending money to try and protect me and save me. Yet, I was still listening to ED. I was a burden and I wanted that to stop and I thought the best way, while still trying to get into recovery, was to do IOP. But I missed the bubble that I had been living in and I think most of all, I was missing the relationship I had with my eating disorder.

I had replaced the comfortable feeling I had in my eating disorder with the comfortable bubble at the treatment center. However, when I got out of the treatment center, I had nothing comfortable left, so what was I supposed to do but go back to ED. The comfortable feeling that I felt in my eating disorder was like home and now without it, where was my home? How did I find a new home when I missed the old one so terribly?

Life seemed very confusing at times. I had to function in a world that I was no longer used to and learn to live in a way to which I was not accustom. I had missed my boyfriend so much while I was away but being back was difficult because we had to learn to be physically together again. I always had that voice in the back of my head, telling me that if I got into recovery that he wouldn't want me anymore and then his voice telling me to please get into recovery, so we could have a life together. It was very difficult battling the voices of my boyfriend and ED especially because I loved my boyfriend, and, at the time, I loved my eating disorder too. I went back and forth between living with my brother and his roommate and living at my boyfriend's. It was confusing because in a time when I was trying to find a home, I was living in two homes and feeling out of a home within myself.

Three evenings a week I spent in a different kind of home, intensive outpatient therapy. For those three nights a week, I would sit in a few rooms with girls and women who think similarly to me. We would listen to the therapists, talk about our feelings, and eat dinner together. Sometimes, we played games to try and make the meals easier to deal with; to think about something other than the task at hand. I found IOP to be a complete change from residential. When the therapists realized that I was using symptoms again, we all decided that it was best for me to enter day treatment. Day treatment meant that 5 days a week I spent my mornings and afternoons with a new group of girls and women; new thoughts and new feelings, except my own; those weren't changing.

It is hard to describe how my thoughts were making me feel. It was like there was still a haze over my eyes and nothing in life was clear; almost like I just couldn't see the world properly. I had almost tunnel vision. It was like I was walking around with my eyes closed expecting to still be able to get around the same way. I had moments of happiness, even some moments when food was involved. I wrestled with my fear foods and overcame all but one. Fear foods for me are foods that made me collapse in anxiety. I couldn't be in the same vicinity as them, and for one particular food, I couldn't be in the same building as the food. If I knew that food was there, I had to leave. For some of my other fear foods, being around them made my heart beat really fast, my hands sweat, my stomach hurt, my head get dizzy and I couldn't think straight. It was almost like an allergic reaction. Then the tears would come, and I would have to leave. My boyfriend helped me slowly get out of my shell and learn that foods won't hurt me and that they can even be enjoyable if I let them.

One of my fear foods was steak, and I remember the first night that I tried to eat a steak. My boyfriend and I were out to dinner with his brother and his brother's girlfriend at the time. It was steak night at the restaurant. They had steaks the length of my forearm that were ten dollars and were supposed to be the best steaks I would ever eat. I remember cutting up the steak into small pieces and taking the first bite. Part of me wanted to admit that it was delicious, but that voice in my head was telling me all the horrible things it always told me. I remember sitting there feeling like I was going to cry. My heart was racing. This was it, I thought.

I kept it together and did the best that I could with all the thoughts running through my head. I didn't finish the steak, mostly because my ED told me that if I finished it that my boyfriend wouldn't love me anymore and my relationship would end. After my boyfriend went to sleep that night, I sat on the floor of the bathroom. I didn't purge, but I wanted to. I believed that because I ate the steak, a little piece of the love he had for me had died and a little piece of myself had fallen away. ED wasn't happy. I had eaten that steak and ED wasn't happy. I wasn't getting it out of my system. I kept it in. I won a battle. It didn't feel as good as you may think.

It is hard to believe that people were still sticking around for me. I was definitely luckier than a lot of the girls that I met in treatment. Yet I still felt like nothing was good enough because I didn't get away with what I wanted to do. My boyfriend had a rule that I couldn't close the bathroom door if I had to go to the bathroom after a meal. At 21, I wasn't trusted by anyone in my life. It made me so angry. Even now, I know there is still not a lot of trust in my life when it comes to ED. I'll get asked frequently, "Did you eat?" or told, "make sure you eat" and it makes me crazy because at 29, you shouldn't be reminded of those things. Sometimes, I have the thoughts that remind me that I am in this position because I put myself there. That is my logical mind. I have a logical mind and an ED mind which usually I can separate.

My logical mind tells me that I don't deserve their trust because my disease causes me to lie or keep secrets. My ED mind makes me think that it is wrong for me to not be trusted. I want to be trusted so that I can use my symptoms in peace when I am not in recovery. This was the same feeling I had back then as well. I just wanted to be able to do what I wanted, even though I knew that it was dangerous. I remembered what the endoscopy pictures looked like.

I've spent so much of my life trying to get everyone's approval that during those times when I lost everyone's trust, it was as if I failed even more than I already had. I don't believe when people say, you can't be perfect. I just know that it is something that I will never be. I read a quote once that said, "you are the perfect you. No one can do it better." I wonder, is that really true? Coming back from treatment and being placed back into care made me feel different. I felt like if someone had the opportunities that I had; if she had my family and my upbringing, she would be able to be me better than me. She wouldn't have fallen into ED's traps. She wouldn't have let a stupid boy control her and make her hate herself. Other me would have been successful by then.

Until recently, I can't remember a time that I didn't have that haze over my eyes. Colors were dimmer than I was told; nothing looked happy. Things could look bright, but colors weren't happy colors. The way that I viewed the world was as if my eyes had been dilated and there was just a blur. I could just see shapes. Sometimes, when I was in treatment, I felt as if I was bringing the other girls down because of my haze. I think I had this mentality while being there that because I couldn't find a way to stay in recovery that meant that no one could. I didn't say that out loud and I didn't believe that. I believe that anyone can get into recovery, but only if it is something that the person really wants. I am a prime example of someone who got into recovery for someone else and when that person left, recovery ended. When he walked out of my life in 2015, everything felt like it was crumbling. As it crumbled down, my recovery went with it. I didn't realize how important it was to get into recovery for yourself until that happened.

During the days of IOP, I think a part of me believed that it didn't matter entirely what your reasons for recovery were, as long as you got into recovery and stopped using symptoms. We were told in treatment that in order to get into recovery you need to believe in recovery and want to stop using symptoms; that it had to be for yourself and no one else. I listened to that, but I don't think I internalized it enough because every time I got into recovery or made an attempt it was for someone else. Recovery wasn't a place that I could find a home. The longer I spent in and out of treatment, the more attempts I made at recovery, the more I felt like I was being pushed further away from finding a home. It wasn't until years later that I found a place that felt like home, but even that didn't last. Nothing lasts…

Chapter 10

I'm standing naked at the mirror
Aware of the feeling of the breeze from the fan on my
skin.
I feel the tears roll down my cheeks as they gaze at the
reflection staring back at me.
So many imperfections; too many curves and roads to
different locations, all ending up at the same destination…
the center of my body; the center of my problem.
All that weighs here in the epicenter determines my worth.
It is here that I learn why I will never be enough.
I collapse to the ground feeling my body convulse, not
being able to hold back the tears or the bile coming up
from my throat.
I heave giving nothing as I have nothing to give, but still
feeling the pain as I realize that no matter what I do or
what I change…
I will never be enough.

You can tell a lot about people through their eyes. You can tell by the glassy, watery look if they have been crying. You can tell by the shape sometimes if they are angry. The eyes are said to be the gateway to the soul, but maybe, the eyes are a gateway to the heart. It is the feelings inside of you that are being shown through your eyes. For people like me, my eyes show my feelings in a different way. My eyes change colors. When I have been crying or I am sad, my eyes turn blue; sometimes so blue that they look like crystals with the sea inside of them. Other times, like when I am angry, my eyes turn so green, it is like a spring meadow overthrowing my eyes; a darker meaning and a ferocious storm on the horizon ready to swallow up anyone that gets in its way. My eyes hide nothing, if you pay close enough attention. My eyes speak out for ED. They always have. It has always been interesting to me how as I get older, ED still stays the same. He looks the same. His words sound the same. He doesn't really learn any new ways to torment me; doesn't tell me anything new or anything that I don't already know. The way his thoughts come through my eyes are always the same; blue and green mixed into a strange grey like the ocean that has been chopped up with seaweed. It shows my mind that has been chopped up by ED. The only thing that changes about him is his voice. My subconscious likes to change the sound of his voice to someone who matters at the time so that I can hear all the cruel thoughts in their voice like they are the ones saying it. ED can be very persuasive. When I was just getting out of IOP, or more like when I dropped out of IOP, ED took on my boyfriend's voice. It was ED telling me that I was fat and worthless. Now that I am older, and I feel worse about myself, he has taken on the voice of someone I care deeply for but can never have. When ED tells me I am disgusting and not worth being loved, it is his voice telling me that all the things I hate about myself are the reasons he will never want me. It is these insecurities that make me feel like it isn't because of anything other than the way I look; that he doesn't want me because he can't be attracted to me. I believe he used to be, but ED's voice continuously reminds me that the lack of affection means that without ED he probably wouldn't even want to be near me.

Life with ED is so painful. There are some moments when it feels so unbearable and the only option is to just give up. I spend so much time fighting to just get by and then I fall backwards a few steps and have to start fighting even harder all over again. It is tiring and sometimes just doesn't feel like it is worth it. Fighting doesn't always seem the viable option. Some days, it feels like fighting is the last thing I want to do. When I have relapsed over the years, it feels as though fighting, like recovery, is just not within my grasp. I can see it, but I can't feel it or touch it. It taunts me quietly with my logical voice saying I could do it, I could fight, but ED jumps in with why? Why fight? Why push so hard to have something that isn't going to change the situation. ED makes me believe that the only way to make someone want me is to let him be in control. I am nothing without ED. For me, nothing will ever work out, so the only thing I have left is to be in this dysfunctional relationship with ED.

Life with ED is exhausting. Not just because the lack of nutrition makes me sleepy, but because some nights I lay awake and just rub my stomach. I think part of me wishes that if I rub enough and push down enough that maybe some of the fat will go away. I do this at night. I do this in the morning. I even catch myself doing it sometimes at work. I just rub down my stomach in the hopes that it will be smaller the next time I do it. Even when I am doing this, I still keep a smile on my face in the presence of other people. I pretend that everything is okay and that I am not wishing that I was wearing something else or was hidden behind a pillow. I fake it until maybe one day I may make it. It is exhausting pretending everything is okay; pretending that I don't hate myself as much as I do. Sometimes, it feels exhausting just for the fact that I spend so much time lying to everyone that I am okay; lying to myself and saying that I am okay. I don't mean to lie to everyone, but how else am I supposed to live my life with ED? As I have gotten older and relapsed so many times, I have come to the realization that maybe I am not supposed to have a life without ED.

My ED determines my worth along with those who deem me not worthy. I feel the pain crush on top of my chest, wondering why if people see me differently than how I see myself, why am I not enough? I try everything to stop the pain. Some people say that I don't; that because I don't escape from certain situations that I am causing the pain, but my solution is what they see as the problem. ED protects me from the problem. ED is my battle armor, not the battle. I remember when there was a time when ED was this war that I was fighting, my team of soldiers off to the rescue to save me from myself. No one is saving me now. I don't need any saving.

Chapter 11

"Since learning of her eating disorder and the damage
done to her body, each day I worry that it will be her last
day, that ED will win. I wonder if she will make it through
the day."

— *Jeff Oppenheim (dad)*

After a period of time, it became apparent that it was best that I be closer to my parents, so I left New York, my brother and my boyfriend and moved back to Florida. Not living in New York was strenuous on the relationship with my boyfriend, so we agreed to just be friends. That was not all that was hard about being back in Florida.

Returning home was difficult because I felt as though I was always being watched. Going to the bathroom after meals meant that I had eyes watching me as I went and questions when I returned. I had therapy sessions every week and friends constantly checking in to see if I wanted to go out for meals as if they really wanted to eat with me every day. It was as if everyone was ganging up on me to make sure I was doing what I was "supposed to be doing." ED was annoyed. I was annoyed. We were fed up. ED would try and convince me of things that I could do. I felt like a piece of me was missing every time I put food in my body. I wasn't happy. I missed the life that I had but it wasn't something that was within my grasp because I wasn't making good decisions. I proved this over and over again.

My boyfriend, now friend, started seeing someone else. I hated it. One night, he told me he was going over to her house and staying with her. I was out with a friend and the overwhelming sadness that I felt because he was starting a new relationship made it impossible to hold down any food, so I purged. After that, I started feeling so sick that I had my friend take me home. I didn't sleep that night because I felt as if my chest was ripping apart and I couldn't breathe. I didn't tell him what I did, but I did tell him of the pain I was in. When I couldn't take the pain anymore, my dad, who hates hospitals, conquered his fear, and took me to the hospital.

Test after test, IV bag after IV bag, and finally the conclusion. I was having a flare-up of my esophagitis. My purging had hurt me. ED had hurt me and in turn I had hurt my dad. I remember laying in the hospital bed in pain and as the morphine washed over me, the last thing I saw before I fell asleep was my dad looking at me and the worry in his blue eyes. His little girl had done it again. This was the first time he had seen me like this. It was always my mom's burden or my boyfriend who had to handle the hospital visits. This was the first time for my dad and the reality of the eating disorder and its toll on me hit my father so hard. My heart began to hurt as much as my chest and throat. I had let him down as I had continued to let my mom and everyone else down.

They released me from the hospital with medication to help heal the damage I had caused, and I decided that day that I wouldn't purge anymore. To me, it was the purging that was causing all of the anxiety and all the damage, not anything else. So, if I stopped the purging, everything would be okay. I wanted so badly for everything to be okay, but I was terrified what that meant for my relationship with ED.

I stayed in Florida for a little while longer, proving that I could live a life without ED or at least with minimal symptom use. I spent my time with my friends and my family for a while until I decided that it was in New York with my boyfriend was where I belonged. Once again, I packed up my belongings and moved back to New York. We reconciled our relationship and it felt so good to be back. Unfortunately, lurking in the shadows was ED just waiting for something to happen so that I could run back to my symptoms; so that I could run back to the relationship that had carried me for so long.

Memories of a Mother

I did not think my feelings of guilt could get worse. That is, until Jeff called to tell me he was taking Aly to the hospital. He described what was going on and how she was feeling, and I spoke with her for just a few moments. The decision to take her to the hospital was a good one, but I was in Baltimore. There was no way that I could be by her side, hold her hand, wipe her tears, and try to help make the pain and misery go away. This time, those challenges were left to Jeff.

Throughout the long day, Jeff called me, or I called him. Thankfully, the morphine allowed Aly to rest and get the sleep she desperately needed. Unfortunately, they do not make drugs for parents whose children are suffering with eating disorders. There are no drugs, no panacea to stop the worry, the anxiety, and the fear. Instead, we pray. Each in his or her own way, we pray and look to God to help our precious baby survive this episode and find her way back into recovery. I know that day and the night before were horrible for Jeff because, until then, the face of her eating disorder had been hidden from him. He knew of her struggles, but nothing can prepare you for seeing the anguish and the pain on your child's face. Now ED, long in the shadows of all of our lives had even consumed our entire family.

Chapter 12

From before she was born, I have prayed each day
That God would protect this precious gift, come what may.
That she would grow up and be healthy and strong
And that I would be able to teach her right from wrong.

Since the moment of her birth I have been full of fears
I have worried about her and shed millions of tears.
When she was young the problems were small
But as she aged, along came ED, a shadow, a wall.

ED consumed by precious child so fast
We did not see the signs, until too much time had passed.
Aly had become so sick and was in such pain
She had become so thin and no weight could she gain.

I look back on those years, the good times and bad.
And think of all of the things that made me so sad.
But then I remember each trip to England she made
Where she found happiness and was no longer afraid.

Phyllis Oppenheim, 2020

"Our doubts are traitors and make us lose the good we oft might win by fearing to attempt."
— William Shakespeare

The only place that had felt like home was when I visited England for a few weeks. It was an international summer school program for Shakespeare; similar to what I would think Shakespeare boot camp would be like if there was such a thing. I was in a world where for the first time I felt like I belonged, and I wasn't just the odd person out. I got to spend all my days studying and talking about my greatest passion with people that understood the same language as me. For the first time in my life, I didn't feel that anyone was judging me or thought I was weird because of how much I loved Shakespeare. They loved his works just as much! I didn't feel I was just the sick girl when I was in England. Life in England was so different and fun. I enjoyed my classes even if sometimes I didn't understand them.

I've always had doubts about my abilities. I don't know if it is because of the eating disorder or just my lack of confidence, but I have always doubted what I am capable of and what I am worth. I don't think I am worth anything. No matter how much I have done and how much education I get, the same things always matter more to me. ED. I know that it may not look like it. As I have heard before, "you don't look like you have an eating disorder" or my favorite, "if you don't eat, how do you still weigh so much?" It is things like this that make me want to give into ED even more. I am not worth anything because I cannot do anything right. If I can't succeed in my own disease, how am I supposed to succeed in anything at all?

There are times in the midst of my disease, during times when there is no recovery in the near future, that it isn't the positive things that give me a sense of accomplishment. During these times, I won't feel guilty for using symptoms, but rather proud, as though I achieved something. I'll feel disappointed and that I failed by eating or going a period of time without using symptoms. I get confused within my head and my body begins doing things without my mind's consent. I look at the Shakespeare quote that is the title of this chapter and at certain times it resonates with my eating disorder and my ED thoughts. I tremble with the thought that my ED could manage to use my greatest passion to further its evil plot. It seems the only thing that I attempt to do is perfect my eating disorder. Going to England and doing these Shakespeare programs were the first things I had done to try and counter my ED thoughts. I tried to not let the fear of failure or not being good enough stop me from doing something that I knew I would love.

During my time in England, everything seemed to make sense to me, except for one thing. ED was still there. I was so happy to be in England each summer and to be studying something that mattered so much to me, but even with that, I still could not get rid of my ED thoughts. I felt as though if I found a "home," it still wouldn't be enough because ED would still be there. It made me feel like ED was my home.

My first summer that I spent in Cambridge was a whirlwind of parties and drinking and men and traveling.

ED thrived on the poor decisions I made and loved how down I felt on myself because of the decisions I was making. If I drank too much, I would throw up and ED would commend me on the weight, he thought I'd lose. If a man hurt me, ED would tell me not to eat because it would make the pain go away. My first summer was a magical summer for ED and yet I didn't even notice that I was having a problem. I was in a drunken haze in England or high in Amsterdam or making out in Paris, so thinking about what food was or was not in my system was not an option. My first summer, although in some ways liberating and fun, caused tremendous damage. When I returned, I was in terrible pain and it was then that I learned of the damage ED and I had done to my body.

While spending my second summer at Cambridge, I first set foot in the place that truly felt like home. It was one of the happiest moments of my life and an entire day when ED didn't make an appearance. This was the day that I visited Stratford-Upon-Avon. No place in the world had ever felt more like home for me than when I rode into town. I rode past the welcome sign and a smile went across my face. Tears came into my eyes as a wave of feelings washed over me. I'd never felt this feeling before. It was like I had been there before and yet it was all so new. We traveled around the town. We went to the theatre and saw *Macbeth*. Everything about that town felt so perfect to me and although I only had one day there to visit, it was a day that I will always cherish because it was a day that even ED couldn't ruin. It was the day I knew I would find a way to live there. I had finally found where I belonged.

The rest of my second trip to England was spent thinking about how I was going to find a way to live in England. I loved it so much there. I didn't use symptoms the rest of the trip, even when I was with my friend in London. I don't know if it was a conscious decision or just something that happened, but ED decided to hide the rest of the time there and let me enjoy the feeling of belonging for the first time in my life. It was the first nice thing ED had ever done for me.

Years later, I found my way back to Stratford and it was everything that I wanted it to be. When I crossed into town and saw the sign welcoming me back, I felt the wave wash over me again and for the second time in my life, I knew, I was where I belonged.

Chapter 13

I look at myself in the mirror
Each angle, turning side to side to see if maybe one
side makes me feel better.
Pulling my shirt in; sucking in my stomach to make myself
believe I can be thin again.
Nothing is good enough.
Then tears roll down my face when
I realize the cold truth…
I will never be good enough.

__Hide your eyes darling; people can see your heart through them.__

– Anonymous

Dear Diary,

There are some moments when I look in the mirror, I feel like I am still looking at that scared, little girl wishing to be thin like the other girls. Now I am wishing to be thin, beautiful, and successful like the other girls; constantly comparing myself to people wondering where I went wrong and why I can't be who I want to be. I look at girls like the ones I constantly compare myself to and wonder what path they took that I wasn't offered so that they could become so successful. This girl is pretty and talented and successful. She would be my competition if there was ever a chance that I could compete against her. Without even trying she would wipe the floor with me in all departments. I look at girls like her and all I feel is that at least I have success in my ED. OH WAIT! No, I don't. I'm not thin enough; I weigh too much; I eat too frequently. I cannot even be successful in my own disease.

Life with ED is awful, but life in the other parts of my mind are sometimes much worse. Lately, ED will at least try and tell me some nice things, I think just to try and counter the thoughts my "logical" mind has been having. It is intriguing as ED is usually the mean thoughts and yet it is the ED voice that is keeping me balanced. I feel crazy with the two sides of my brain at war with one another. I may be able to hide the pain from most of the people in my life; put a smile on and pretend that everything is okay, but it isn't. I want to be happy, I think. I am not really sure what would bring me happiness. I used to think that ED brought me happiness, but how can a disease that actively tries to make you sick, make you happy. I have thoughts that if I was thinner or beautiful (even pretty), if I was smarter or had better attention to detail, that maybe I'd be a step closer to the girl I dreamt of being when I was little. What is sad is loving someone and seeing that person is successful, pretty and smart and having to come to terms with the fact that it isn't you.

I compare myself to everyone. There are qualities about each girl I see that makes her somehow better than me. Some girls have more qualities than others that make me feel like I am not worthy of love because I am not tall enough, successful enough, confident enough. I guess it comes down to the fact that I don't feel like I am enough.

There are no safe corners in my mind. ED and the sadness have taken them all away. I feel this is part of the disease though. I fight and fight to climb out of this hole; this abyss, called ED. Some days I climb higher and can see that little bit of freedom. I can see the smiling, proud faces at the top cheering me on. Then something happens, and I can still see those faces, but now there is fear in their eyes as I fall backwards, back into the abyss. My biggest fear is disappointing people and yet the deeper I get into my relapse, the more my ED tells me that this is more important. It is more important to be thin and try and feel beautiful than my fear of disappointing anyone around me.

My logical mind is losing the battle, except for one thing; one person. I am terrified of disappointing the man in my life. I guess it always comes down to a single person.

When I first got treatment, it was a person that got me into recovery. It was that fear of disappointing him that pushed me to do what I was scared of doing. Now it isn't that I am scared of recovery, it is that I don't want it. However, this person keeps me from falling over the edge entirely. I won't use symptoms around him. My heart leads the way and gives my mind a small break when I am around him. Sometimes, even when I am not hungry, and my mind is screaming at me to not put anything in my body; when I am feeling so nauseated by my body, I will still eat… for him. That is the best I can offer right now.

My heart wishes that I could give more. It wishes that this wasn't so difficult and that at times, I would just listen to it and move forward. But I can't just do things to make him happy. I do a lot of things to make him happy, to make him proud, but this just isn't one of them. I can't offer him my recovery. Everyone leaves so when he does, if I give him my recovery, then I won't know what to do anymore when he is gone. I know that my recovery has to be for me, so I can't put it out there for someone else, no matter how badly I would like to sometimes. Unfortunately, it just isn't something that I want. I think that these dark times present the first time that my heart breaks for me. I feel sad at times, and the only reason is because I am sad for myself. I am sad that I can't bring myself to be in recovery; that I can't make me like myself. I am sad that I have such little confidence that I can barely spend a few hours in my own company.

You see, the problem with ED is not necessarily just the thoughts and feelings that come out of it, but the reaction to them. The feeling that you can't look in the mirror, shower, get dressed, be intimate or even walk outside without hearing that voice control you. I don't feel functional. I don't feel happy. I feel alone in my thoughts and nothing can pull me out. ED is something that I live with every day. He has been there from the time I was 10, wanting to fit in with the other girls to even now wanting to compare to those that mean more to the world than I do.

I wish I meant more. I wish I was more. I wish I was enough.

Sincerely,
Never enough Penguin

Chapter 14

I'm standing naked at the mirror
Aware of the feeling of the breeze from the fan on my
skin.
I feel him leer at me and I kneel.
No words are needed between us anymore for me to know
what is expected of me.
I submit to his needs with the sadistic thought that I feed
off his joy.
I cry for the girl I once was;
The girl that I can't remember but know once existed.
I cry, but yet change nothing.
He leers, and I obey.
No words are spoken as I rise and look into my blood shot
eyes.
I go into my room and curl into a ball until the pain
subsides.
I cry, but he wins.
He always wins.

There is no glory, only pain.

Dear Diary,

At times, throughout this book and throughout my life, it seems like I am glorifying my eating disorder. That is very common. It is hard not to glorify something that I have spent most of my life thinking of as my best friend. The problem with that is there is no glory. There is pain and harshness and sadness. ED is not my best friend. ED is a shadow that follows and haunts. The sadistic, proud feeling that I get is not me; it is ED taking over my mind. To be completely honest, I am writing this chapter as quickly as I can because it is in a moment of clarity when I feel logical and not driven by my ED thoughts.

Today I used every symptom I have ever used. I restricted, I purged, and I took a laxative. To be honest, I have never done this before. Usually I will choose one symptom at a time per day and go forth with that, but today is a different type of day. Today is a new day where ED has been so unbearable and so loud that I needed to use as many symptoms as possible to keep the thoughts from taking over my head. I have had a headache for days with the shouting and demeaning thoughts that have been going through my head and yet I have had a smile on my face. The smile isn't mine. ED has taken over all of me to the point where I don't know where I end, and he begins. When the thoughts have consumed me, I have found excuses to tell those around me if they ask what is wrong. I am built up of excuses and they work because everyone wants to believe that I am okay. I am not okay.

My head is pounding. My stomach is pulsing. My throat is burning, and my pulse is racing. Nothing about me feels okay and if someone were to take a second and look deep into my eyes likc they were searching for something, they'd know. ED has taken so much from me and yet I cannot seem to stop giving him the power to continue. I can't stand the screaming. I want it to go away, but late at night when the voice finally stops, I feel so lonely. I hate the loneliness. It amuses me when people tell me that I stay in situations with people so that I am not lonely. It isn't the loneliness of people that scares me. It is the loneliness of being rid of the voice in my head that makes me scared and for some reason with certain people in my life, ED has more room to roam.

When I get into these logical moments, I think that I want a life without ED. I can remember what it was like when I wasn't sad or breaking all the time. I can remember what it was like to not feel raw inside my stomach or pain inside my throat. It amazes me how different life was, just one year ago. It amazes me how different life always is when I go from life without ED to life with ED. It feels like everything around me stays the same, but little pieces of the haze come back. It has been one year since I felt the sick, hunger feeling and for the first time in so long did nothing about it. It has been one year since I welcomed my dolly back from the drawer with open arms; since I welcomed the lover back with apologies.

Each day with ED feels like a year in itself. Time goes quickly and slowly all at once and at the end of each day in whichever bed I am going to sleep, ED is there wishing me sweet dreams and that he will speak to me tomorrow like a lover does when separated only by distance. ED is the type of lover that has your heart in one hand, slowly tracing the arteries with his thumb and his other hand wrapped tightly around your neck; looking lovingly into your eyes as he shows you his control.

Sincerely,
Me

I've learned more as I have grown up about the haze that covers my life. As I got older, I was diagnosed with bipolar disorder and as soon as I was placed on the proper medication the haze began to dissipate. The haze that was covering my world was my depression and as soon as I was medicated it was like I was literally seeing a different world. ED doesn't like this though because he thrives on the fear. He loved the haze. That was his vacation home. He still finds places to hide even when the haze is gone, but during the time of the haze he was much more active. He always finds a way to control. He does not need haze or depression to take control of me. It takes all of my strength and all of my courage; like that of a victim taking control over her attacker. I have to fight back, and it is never easy. ED dominates. ED controls and leaves pieces of me in his wake. I need to fight back. I want to fight back, but I am scared. What would life be like without him? What would I be without him? Would I be without him?

Chapter 15

I stared at myself in the mirror trying to talk myself out of
doing it;
Ignoring the sad music that made its way out of my phone
speakers.

It had been weeks since I gave into that demand of the
demon.
I looked at my eyes and I could see his leer that told me
that no matter how badly I argued,
He would win.

A tear rolled down my face and a "no" escaped my lips as
I got to the ground.
I stared in as if I was staring into a tunnel with a dark
nothingness at the end of it.

I tried to pay attention to the lyrics and ignore the almost
involuntary motion of my arm and fingers, but the jolt
came quickly this time and I couldn't help but give into
the demands.

I heard a sound of cheer from the bastard in my head.
I heard the praise.
I stared at myself in the mirror and with that lonely
teardrop, I smiled.

Dear Diary,

Sometimes, I lay down and fall asleep and in the comfort of my dreams, I remember a time when I felt confident and beautiful. When I wake up, I wonder if I was dreaming of someone else's life. In the light of day, I can never remember the times that plague me in my dreams. When my eyes are open, there are times when all I can think of is, will I ever have a body of which I am proud? Is having confidence at this age even possible if you do not have it now? Going through life, with this monster on my shoulder, makes it difficult to hear any of the other voices that try and scream into my ears in order to battle the demon.

When did life become filled with new ways to bring yourself down? You're too fat; you're too tall; you're too short; your breasts are too big; too small. Everywhere you go, you are thrown into a world of posters and magazines telling you how you should lose weight, that you should lose weight; that the only way that your man won't cheat on you is if you are a size 2. Why is life so determined to be about what we look like rather than who we are? And if times tried to change, would people accept it, or would women continue to bring themselves down and try to change for love?

I woke up this morning and rolled over thinking that things could be easy; thinking that maybe I didn't care after all that I am not a size 2. But then my eyes opened. The sun came in the window and the room appeared to be just as I left it before I went to sleep. A handsome man was lying beside me, my room smelled of the wax melts I had burned the other day. Everything seemed to be normal… except for me. I stared up at the ceiling and all I could see was the face of my doctor the other day, when I told her that I wanted to lose weight. Kept seeing that look on her face that the demon had taken something else from me; my ability to lose weight. I could tell that she was hesitant to even try a weight loss program with me, but she was willing to give it a shot if I let the possible meds that she was going to give me be monitored by my mother. I was a child.

When did honesty turn into the new reason to not be trusted? When did telling the truth begin taking away your ability to do things on your own? I walked out of the appointment with an even heavier weight on my shoulder. What would I do if I couldn't lose weight and was stuck like this forever? It's been two days and the weight growing on my shoulders keeps getting heavier. The voice of the monster living in the dark corners of my shadow keeps telling me to just give my old habits a chance and that maybe they would have a different effect this time. Each time it comes closer to mealtime, I begin my battle with the demon. I fight it by asking when we will eat; by taking a bite of foods I know I enjoy. But I am losing my will to continue fighting. I have been fighting for so long and nothing has come of it. I fight to not eat; I fight to eat. I fight to be thin by using symptoms and I fight by trying to be healthy. When did my life become a battle of the demons?

It has now been two days since the masses have grown on my shoulders. Today they took blood as the first of three steps to hopefully getting healthy. The next step is more tests and then we move on to the results and what the plan will be pending the results. This is the plan that helped my mother, so logically it should mean that it will help me too. However, nothing in my life has been logical. Nothing has made sense since the first day that I looked in the mirror and cried because of what was looking back at me. It is strange when I think back on those times. Growing up, tearing up every time I looked in a mirror and now, I am an adult who gazes at this body, not knowing who she is. Looking at and wondering how I hated my old body, the phrase, "the grass is always greener" has never proven truer for me then now.

I used to be able to look in the mirror and see beauty in my face. I could look at my eyes and see past the holes of despair and see the ocean grey. I could see the shape of my face; the defined jaw line and think that even if I didn't like my body, I at least had a face of which I could be proud. Now the blemishes are more prevalent, the face rounder. The only thing still there are the eyes; still filled with despair and sadness, but still have the ocean grey swimming through them with a storm on the horizon.

Chapter 16

"You wake up every morning to fight the same demons that left you so tired the night before, and that, my love, is bravery."

— Anonymous

I used to think that recovery wasn't possible for me. I would sit in groups with people that achieved greatness in their recovery and thought, "wow! That is amazing, but I will never get there." Recovery was a foreign concept for me because no matter how hard I thought I was trying, I never got past 3 or 4 months. Something would happen that would set me off and I would begin spiraling out of control again and there would be my shadow, grasping my hand to hold me up in the worst kind of way. At age 23, that all changed. I got into recovery and things began to fall into place. My ED didn't feel like it was lurking around every corner as much. I could still hear him sometimes in my head, but he didn't overtake every thought. I could have a meal without his voice over reacting. I could go on a date with my boyfriend and not worry about what ED would think. Life was different for me. I finally knew what life was like without ED.

At 24, I decided that I wanted to pursue my dream of earning a master's degree in England. The only contingency was that, if I were to be accepted, I would have to get approval from my entire treatment team before being allowed to move to England. This was the first time in the life that I could remember that I thought I could actually accomplish a dream I had been dreaming of since I was a little child. I wasn't even supposed to really be alive anymore considering that I had still spent years battling my eating disorder and now I had the opportunity to move across the world and pursue my dream. I was ready to fight and most of all, I was ready to tell ED to go screw himself for good. I had spent so many days and nights trying to sleep as long as possible just so that I didn't have to fight with ED. So many hours with this demon on my shoulder that now it was time to use all the courage I had and separate from what I grew up thinking was my best friend – my only friend.

I submitted my applications for graduate school in September of 2014. I applied to two schools: Cambridge University and the University of Birmingham's Shakespeare Institute. I was told when I graduated undergrad that if I was going to apply to grad school to apply to at least six because more than likely, I wouldn't get in to any or very few. I had one professor tell me that I wasn't good enough to get into any program and I was wasting my time. He tried to break me. He failed because in 2014, I was accepted into the Shakespeare Institute. By the following summer, with my acceptance letter in hand, the approval of my treatment team and one year of recovery under my belt, I was getting ready to move to England to pursue my dream of getting my masters in Shakespeare Studies.

My mom flew over to England with me to help me get settled. She spent a few days, seeing Stratford-Upon-Avon with me and admiring the little town that I was going to call home for the next year. But, on one beautiful misty morning in England, I watched my mom's taxi drive away. I was alone.

At 25 years old, I had gone through so many traumatic experiences in life. I had spent so many years in pain, engulfed in a shadow that I couldn't free myself from. I thought that ED was my friend. I thought that without ED, I would be lost and that no one would want to be around me. But, as I stood in my driveway in England and watched as the taxi got smaller; smelled the dew in the air of the town I'd dreamt of for years that was now my home, I realized that ED was never my friend, best or otherwise. He was my shadow and as I took a walk to the River Avon, I finally felt free.

Memories of a Mother

I had gone to Baltimore for work the beginning of September 2014, and Aly took the bus down from New York to spend the day and night with me. I will always remember, sitting with her in the hotel room, watching as she finished her application to the Shakespeare Institute. We had talked so much about the conditions that would exist, if she were accepted. What she would have to do in order to go to England to study. She knew what was at stake and her face positively glowed when she hit SUBMIT. Aly had taken the first step toward her dream of studying in England.

Waiting to learn if she was accepted was agonizing for all of us but, of course, mostly for her. When she finally received the letter, she was told that the program she had applied for was not going to happen, but they were putting her into the other program, if she wanted to attend. What an understatement! As it turned out, she was accepted into the program that she had wanted all along. Now the difficult part was to begin.

Aly knew that we would not permit her to go to England unless her entire recovery team believed that she was healthy enough to go. She wanted this so badly and, thankfully, she did everything that she had to do in order to get the "all clear." I cannot imagine the inner strength that it took for her to get into recovery but, for the first time, recovery was possible. And, maybe for the first time, this recovery would be for her, no one else.

One year to the day of her submitting the application to the Institute, Aly and I boarded the plane for London. She was so happy and excited. Everything had fallen into place. She was, according to her team, in recovery, and well enough to go. The VISA and finances worked out. She had a flat in Stratford-Upon-Avon and, from the emails, a wonderful landlady.

We traveled from London by bus to the bus station in a town near Stratford-Upon-Avon and then took a cab to her flat. My first impression of this quaint town was that it was, for Aly, home. Her flat was across the street and a mere four doors away from the home where Shakespeare was born! Those few days we spent together in England were filled with amazing times, walking through the plaza, walking to the Trinity Church and seeing where Shakespeare is buried, going to Anne Hathaway's Cottage (where she would end up working the entire year she was in England), spending time talking and laughing. At times, the heartache and worries brought about by her eating disorder disappeared. We were just mom and Aly, just as we were when she was younger, before ED took such control of her.

She was worried about being in England for the high holidays and staying with a wonderful observant family in Birmingham. For the first time in her life, we would be apart for the holidays and, in recovery, this was the first year she would have to eat on Yom Kippur and not give into ED by fasting. Thankfully, we were able to work that out too as the family was so understanding.

My time in England went by too fast. In what seemed like a blink of an eye, it was time for me to return to the States. It was time to say goodbye. Aly and I had agreed that it made no sense for her to travel back to London with me. I had to leave early in the morning, take the cab to the bus, the bus to the airport. She had an interview that day for a job with the Shakespeare Birthplace Trust (she got the job). Instead, we called for the cab to be there early in the morning and she helped me bring my bags down. As I hugged my precious baby goodbye, I was once again forced to hold back the tears that I knew would come. We both kept it together long enough to say goodbye. She looked so happy, albeit a bit scared, but sure of herself. This is where she wanted to be. Stratford-Upon-Avon would be her new home and, hopefully, a place where she would find the peace and freedom from ED that she had sought for so long. I looked through the back window of the cab as we pulled away, the tears falling from my eyes. As Aly appeared smaller and smaller the farther away we got, I thanked God for letting her get this far and prayed that ED was finally gone from her life.

He tries to pull me down his path, but I release his hands
and stand at the crossroads.
I turn and look down the other side and a warm, relaxing
breeze draws me in.

He calls to me with his smooth, seductive voice and I turn
my body, but not my head.
He always controls my body, but this other path, this
breeze is calling to me.

He tries to entice me down his path, but I take a step
towards the opposite.
His face falls.
He tells me the sweet nothings that have kept me his slave
for so many years,
And yet I still look down this unknown path. This
unknown yet welcoming path.

I know this path. I've seen it before.
He screams. This isn't what he wants.

I take another step and then another.
He shouts after me as I chase the wind down this
mysterious path.

I do not know what waits for me down this path.
But, as the warm breeze envelopes me in a hug, I feel a
wave rush over me.

I'm safe.

He can't touch me here and with the crossroads behind
me, I continue my journey into the unknown.

And for the first time, I'm free.

2015

References

[1]Anorexia Nervosa and Associated Disorders. (2018). Retrieved from

http://www.anad.org/education-and-awareness/about-eating-disorders/eating-disorders-statistics/

[2]Anorexia Nervosa and Associated Disorders. (2018). Retrieved from

http://www.anad.org/education-and-awareness/about-eating-disorders/eating-disorders-statistics/

[3]National Institute of Mental Health. (2016). Eating disorders. Retrieved from

https://www.nimh.nih.gov/health/topics/eating-disorders /index.shtml #part_145412

[4]Anorexia Nervosa and Associated Disorders. (2018). Retrieved from

http://www.anad.org/education-and-awareness/about-eating-disorders/eating-disorders-statistics/